# food & diet counter
Complete nutritional facts for every diet!

**Dr Wynnie Chan**    hamlyn

First published in Great Britain in 2003 by Hamlyn,
a division of Octopus Publishing Group Ltd,
2–4 Heron Quays, London E14 4JP

ISBN-13: 978-0-600-60709-0
ISBN-10: 0-600-60709-7

A CIP catalogue record for this book is available
from the British Library

Printed and bound in Spain

10 9 8 7 6 5 4 3 2

Nutrient information has been calculated using data from the
UK Food Nutrient Databank which is available from The Food
Standards Agency (FSA). Some values have been estimated
based on similar foods.
The information in this book is intended only as a guide to
following a healthy diet. People with special dietary
requirements of any kind should consult appropriate medical
professionals before changing their diet.

# CONTENTS

Whether you want to lose just a few kilograms or rather more, eating healthily is vital. This does not mean cutting out all of your favourite treats completely, just eating them in moderation. If you're not enjoying your food, you are less likely to stick to your diet and exercise regime.

Losing weight doesn't just mean that you'll have more energy and feel better about yourself, it also decreases the risk of developing various ailments, including diabetes, hypertension, coronary heart disease, stroke, respiratory problems, gallstones and some cancers.

## What is a healthy weight?

The formula used to establish whether a person is too thin, the right weight, fat or obese is called the Body Mass Index (BMI). This is a simple measurement of weight against height, and can be calculated using the following equation:

$$\frac{\text{weight (kg)}}{\text{height (m) x height (m)}}$$

So, a person weighing 56kg who is 1.5m tall has a BMI of 25:
$56 \div (1.5 \times 1.5) = 25$.
Alternatively:

$$\frac{\text{weight (lb) x 703}}{\text{height (in) x height (in)}}$$

So, the same person, weighing 123lb who is 59 in tall has the same BMI of 25:
$123 \times 703 \div (59 \times 59) = 25$.

BMI RATINGS

| | |
|---|---|
| below 20: | underweight |
| 20–24.9: | normal weight |
| 25–29.9: | overweight |
| 30–39.9: | moderate obesity |
| Over 40: | severe obesity |

## Balanced diets

Including foods from the five food groups means that you are meeting your requirements for nutrients.

THE FIVE GROUPS ARE:

**1 Bread, cereals and potatoes.** This group is rich in starchy carbohydrates and includes breakfast cereals, rice, pasta, noodles, yams and oats and should form the basis of most meals. Foods in this group are rich in insoluble fibre, calcium, iron and B vitamins, which are needed to keep your gut, bones and blood healthy. Try to eat wholegrain, wholemeal or high-fibre versions of breads and cereals.

## 2 Fruits and vegetables.

These are important sources of antioxidants such as vitamin C and beta-carotene (vegetable vitamin A), which protect us from cancers and heart disease. They are also rich in soluble fibre, which helps lower blood cholesterol. Try to include five portions of different fruits and vegetables in your diet each day, whether fresh, frozen, canned, dried or juiced.

### A portion of fruit equals:

■ 1 slice of pineapple, grapefruit, melon or watermelon, or half a mango or papaya
■ 1 whole apple, avocado, banana, orange, peach or pear
■ 2 small apricots, clementines, figs, kiwi fruit, passion fruit, plums, satsumas or tomatoes
■ 1 cupful of berries, cherries or grapes
■ 3 tablespoons stewed or canned apples, apricots, fruit cocktail, pears, peaches or pineapple, or fresh fruit salad
■ 1 tablespoon dried apricots, bananas, cranberries, dates, figs, papaya, pineapple, raisins or sultanas
■ 1 (150ml/5floz) glass of fruit juice (not fruit drinks or fruit squashes)

### A portion of vegetables equals:

■ 2 tablespoons broccoli, brussels sprouts, cabbage, cauliflower, radishes, turnip, swede, chard, winter greens, kale, pak choi, rocket, romaine lettuce, spinach, aubergine, carrots, green beans, mushrooms, onions, peas, peppers or squash
■ half a cupful of alfalfa, baked beans, beansprouts, sprouting broccoli, black beans, chickpeas, kidney beans, lentils or soya beans
■ 1 dessert bowl of salad
■ 1 (150ml/5floz) glass of carrot, beetroot or wheatgrass juice

## 3 Milk and dairy foods.

These are excellent sources of calcium, protein and vitamins A and B12, essential for maintaining the health of bones, skin and blood. Include a couple of reduced-fat servings from this food group each day.

## 4 Meat, fish and alternatives.

The main nutrients supplied by this food group include iron, protein, B vitamins, zinc and magnesium, which help to maintain healthy blood and an efficient immune system. Choose at most two servings of lean red meat, fish, chicken, nuts, turkey, eggs, be or pulses. The last two are great protein alternatives, as is tofu, wh is also a good source of calcium.

**5** Foods containing sugar or fat. Minimize your intake of savoury snacks, biscuits, cakes, crisps, pastries, sweets, chocolate, pies, butter and carbonated drinks, as these will hinder your efforts to lose weight.

## Watch the fat

Gram for gram, fat has more than twice as many calories as protein and carbohydrates:

| Calories per gram | kcal | kJ |
|---|---|---|
| fat | 9 | 37 |
| protein | 4 | 17 |
| carbohydrate | 3.75 | 16 |

Foods with high levels of fat tend to be low in fibre and are not filling, so we eat more of these than high-carbohydrate foods. This raises the calorie intake even farther. Most of us should eat at least 25g (1oz) less fat a day.

GOOD FAT, BAD FAT

All fats will increase your weight if you eat too much, but not all raise the risk of developing disease. There are three types of fat: saturated, monounsaturated and polyunsaturated. The former raise levels of 'bad' cholesterol in the blood. Cholesterol is carried around

the body by two proteins: low-density lipoprotein (LDL) and high-density lipoprotein (HDL). When levels of LDL cholesterol are raised in the blood, it may be deposited on the blood vessel walls, narrowing them so they become blocked. If blood supply to the heart is interrupted it can lead to a heart attack which in severe cases can be fatal.

HDL is considered good as it carries cholesterol from various parts of the body to the liver where it can be disposed of.

As a general rule, fats that are hard at room temperature will contain the most saturated fat. Cakes, butter, cheese, biscuits, cooking fats, pastries, pies, fatty meat, whole milk and hard margarine provide the most saturated fats in our diets so cut down on these.

The monounsaturated and polyunsaturated fats are found in vegetable oils and fat spreads, and are considered healthier than saturated fats. Replacing the latter with the other versions can lower levels of LDL cholesterol.

Fatty or oily fish like sardines, salmon, mackerel, herring and trout contain polyunsaturated fats called omega-3 fats. These help to protect against heart disease. We should eat a serving of oily fish each week.

## Guideline Daily Amounts

Guideline Daily Amounts (GDAs) are daily guideline figures recommended by health professionals for intake of calories, fat and saturates for adult women and men. These are average figures and personal requirements will vary with age, weight and levels of activity.

AVERAGE DAILY REQUIREMENT

|  | women | men |
|---|---|---|
| kcal | 2000 | 2500 |
| fat | 70g | 95g |
| saturates | 20g | 30g |

## Dietary Reference Values

Dietary Reference Values (DRVs) are daily recommendations set by the Department of Health for the nutrients considered sufficient for most adults and children in the UK. The table below gives the average daily requirement for protein, carbohydrate and fibre. If you are trying to lose weight, you will need less, and should discuss the exact amounts with your doctor or dietician.

AVERAGE DAILY REQUIREMENT

|  | women | men |
|---|---|---|
| protein | 46g | 56g |
| carbohydrate | 225g | 300g |
| fibre | 18g | 18g |

**How to use this book**
It lists the energy, as kilocalories (kcal) and kilojoules (kJ), fat, saturated fat, protein, carbohydrate and fibre contained in more than 1500 foods. Nutrient values have been expressed as average servings so no calculator is needed.

The information shows where the energy comes from in any food so, if you're on a low-fat, low-carbohydrate diet or have any other special requirements, you can work out exactly how much you can have of any food.

**Note**
The average portion sizes of foods were obtained from *Food Portion Sizes, Second Edition,* HMSO, 1999. This information is based on a) weighed dietary surveys conducted by the Ministry of Agriculture, Fisheries and Food, b) information from manufacturers and c) by weighing numerous samples of foods such as takeaway dishes.

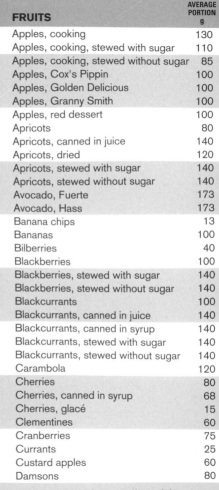

| FRUITS | AVERAGE PORTION g |
|---|---|
| Apples, cooking | 130 |
| Apples, cooking, stewed with sugar | 110 |
| Apples, cooking, stewed without sugar | 85 |
| Apples, Cox's Pippin | 100 |
| Apples, Golden Delicious | 100 |
| Apples, Granny Smith | 100 |
| Apples, red dessert | 100 |
| Apricots | 80 |
| Apricots, canned in juice | 140 |
| Apricots, dried | 120 |
| Apricots, stewed with sugar | 140 |
| Apricots, stewed without sugar | 140 |
| Avocado, Fuerte | 173 |
| Avocado, Hass | 173 |
| Banana chips | 13 |
| Bananas | 100 |
| Bilberries | 40 |
| Blackberries | 100 |
| Blackberries, stewed with sugar | 140 |
| Blackberries, stewed without sugar | 140 |
| Blackcurrants | 100 |
| Blackcurrants, canned in juice | 140 |
| Blackcurrants, canned in syrup | 140 |
| Blackcurrants, stewed with sugar | 140 |
| Blackcurrants, stewed without sugar | 140 |
| Carambola | 120 |
| Cherries | 80 |
| Cherries, canned in syrup | 68 |
| Cherries, glacé | 15 |
| Clementines | 60 |
| Cranberries | 75 |
| Currants | 25 |
| Custard apples | 60 |
| Damsons | 80 |

Unless otherwise stated, fruits are prepared but uncooked.

| ENERGY kcal | ENERGY kJ | FAT g | SATURATED FAT g | PROTEIN g | CARBOHYDRATE g | FIBRE g |
|---|---|---|---|---|---|---|
| 46 | 196 | Trace | Trace | 0 | 12 | 2.1 |
| 81 | 345 | Trace | Trace | 0 | 21 | 1.3 |
| 28 | 117 | Trace | Trace | 0 | 7 | 1.3 |
| 46 | 195 | Trace | Trace | 1 | 11 | 2 |
| 43 | 185 | Trace | Trace | 0 | 11 | 1.7 |
| 45 | 193 | Trace | Trace | 0 | 12 | 1.7 |
| 51 | 217 | Trace | Trace | 0 | 13 | 1.9 |
| 25 | 107 | Trace | Trace | 1 | 6 | 1.4 |
| 48 | 206 | Trace | Trace | 1 | 12 | 1.3 |
| 190 | 809 | 1 | Trace | 5 | 44 | 7.6 |
| 101 | 431 | Trace | Trace | 1 | 26 | 2.2 |
| 38 | 161 | Trace | Trace | 1 | 9 | 2.1 |
| 327 | 1349 | 33 | 6.1 | 4 | 3 | 5.9 |
| 330 | 1362 | 34 | 8.1 | 3 | 3 | 5.9 |
| 66 | 278 | 4 | Trace | 0 | 8 | 0.2 |
| 95 | 403 | 1 | 0.1 | 1 | 23 | 1.1 |
| 12 | 51 | Trace | Trace | 0 | 3 | 0.7 |
| 25 | 104 | Trace | Trace | 1 | 5 | 3.1 |
| 78 | 335 | Trace | Trace | 1 | 19 | 3.4 |
| 29 | 123 | Trace | Trace | 1 | 6 | 3.6 |
| 28 | 121 | Trace | Trace | 1 | 7 | 3.6 |
| 43 | 189 | Trace | Trace | 1 | 11 | 4.3 |
| 101 | 428 | Trace | Trace | 1 | 26 | 3.6 |
| 81 | 353 | Trace | Trace | 1 | 21 | 3.9 |
| 34 | 144 | Trace | Trace | 1 | 8 | 4.3 |
| 38 | 163 | 1 | 0.1 | 1 | 9 | 1.6 |
| 38 | 162 | Trace | Trace | 1 | 9 | 0.7 |
| 48 | 207 | Trace | Trace | 0 | 13 | 0.4 |
| 39 | 159 | Trace | Trace | 0 | 9 | 0 |
| 22 | 95 | Trace | Trace | 1 | 5 | 0.7 |
| 11 | 49 | Trace | Trace | 0 | 3 | 2.3 |
| 67 | 285 | Trace | Trace | 1 | 17 | 0.5 |
| 41 | 178 | Trace | Trace | 1 | 10 | 1.4 |
| 30 | 130 | Trace | Trace | 0 | 8 | 1.4 |

FRUITS

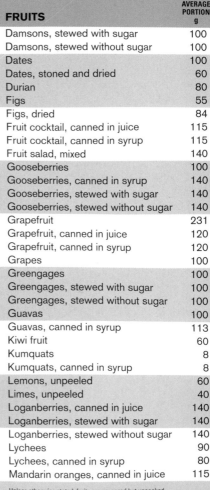

| FRUITS | AVERAGE PORTION g |
|---|---|
| Damsons, stewed with sugar | 100 |
| Damsons, stewed without sugar | 100 |
| Dates | 100 |
| Dates, stoned and dried | 60 |
| Durian | 80 |
| Figs | 55 |
| Figs, dried | 84 |
| Fruit cocktail, canned in juice | 115 |
| Fruit cocktail, canned in syrup | 115 |
| Fruit salad, mixed | 140 |
| Gooseberries | 100 |
| Gooseberries, canned in syrup | 140 |
| Gooseberries, stewed with sugar | 140 |
| Gooseberries, stewed without sugar | 140 |
| Grapefruit | 231 |
| Grapefruit, canned in juice | 120 |
| Grapefruit, canned in syrup | 120 |
| Grapes | 100 |
| Greengages | 100 |
| Greengages, stewed with sugar | 100 |
| Greengages, stewed without sugar | 100 |
| Guavas | 100 |
| Guavas, canned in syrup | 113 |
| Kiwi fruit | 60 |
| Kumquats | 8 |
| Kumquats, canned in syrup | 8 |
| Lemons, unpeeled | 60 |
| Limes, unpeeled | 40 |
| Loganberries, canned in juice | 140 |
| Loganberries, stewed with sugar | 140 |
| Loganberries, stewed without sugar | 140 |
| Lychees | 90 |
| Lychees, canned in syrup | 80 |
| Mandarin oranges, canned in juice | 115 |

Unless otherwise stated, fruits are prepared but uncooked.

| ENERGY kcal | ENERGY kJ | FAT g | SATURATED FAT g | PROTEIN g | CARBOHYDRATE g | FIBRE g |
|---|---|---|---|---|---|---|
| 74 | 316 | Trace | Trace | 0 | 19 | 1.5 |
| 34 | 147 | Trace | Trace | 1 | 9 | 1.6 |
| 124 | 530 | Trace | Trace | 2 | 31 | 1.8 |
| 162 | 691 | 1 | 0.1 | 2 | 41 | 2.4 |
| 109 | 460 | 1 | Trace | 2 | 23 | 3 |
| 24 | 102 | 1 | 0.1 | 1 | 5 | 0.8 |
| 176 | 747 | 1 | Trace | 3 | 41 | 5.8 |
| 33 | 140 | Trace | Trace | 0 | 8 | 1.2 |
| 66 | 281 | Trace | Trace | 0 | 17 | 1.2 |
| 77 | 332 | Trace | Trace | 1 | 19 | 2.1 |
| 40 | 170 | 1 | 0.1 | 1 | 9 | 2.4 |
| 102 | 434 | Trace | Trace | 1 | 26 | 2.4 |
| 76 | 321 | Trace | Trace | 1 | 18 | 2.7 |
| 22 | 92 | Trace | Trace | 1 | 4 | 2.8 |
| 69 | 291 | Trace | Trace | 2 | 16 | 3 |
| 36 | 144 | Trace | Trace | 1 | 9 | 0.5 |
| 72 | 308 | Trace | Trace | 1 | 19 | 0.7 |
| 60 | 257 | Trace | Trace | 0 | 15 | 0.7 |
| 41 | 173 | Trace | Trace | 1 | 10 | 2.1 |
| 81 | 347 | Trace | Trace | 1 | 21 | 1.9 |
| 36 | 155 | Trace | Trace | 1 | 9 | 1.9 |
| 26 | 112 | 1 | Trace | 1 | 5 | 3.7 |
| 68 | 292 | Trace | Trace | 0 | 18 | 3.4 |
| 29 | 124 | Trace | Trace | 1 | 6 | 1.1 |
| 3 | 15 | Trace | Trace | 0 | 1 | 0.3 |
| 11 | 46 | Trace | Trace | 0 | 3 | 0.1 |
| 8 | 36 | 1 | 0.1 | 0 | 1 | 1.7 |
| 4 | 14 | 0 | 0 | 0 | 0 | 1.1 |
| 141 | 601 | Trace | Trace | 1 | 37 | 2.2 |
| 70 | 300 | Trace | Trace | 1 | 18 | 2.8 |
| 20 | 87 | Trace | Trace | 1 | 4 | 2.9 |
| 52 | 223 | Trace | Trace | 1 | 13 | 0.6 |
| 54 | 232 | Trace | Trace | 0 | 14 | 0.4 |
| 37 | 155 | Trace | Trace | 1 | 9 | 0.3 |

| FRUITS | AVERAGE PORTION g |
|---|---|
| Mandarin oranges, canned in syrup | 126 |
| Mangoes | 150 |
| Mangoes, canned in syrup | 105 |
| Mangosteen | 60 |
| Melon, Canteloupe | 150 |
| Melon, Galia | 150 |
| Melon, Honeydew | 200 |
| Mixed peel | 5 |
| Nectarines | 150 |
| Oranges | 160 |
| Papaya | 140 |
| Passion fruit | 60 |
| Peaches | 110 |
| Peaches, canned in juice | 120 |
| Peaches, canned in syrup | 120 |
| Pears, canned in juice | 135 |
| Pears, canned in syrup | 135 |
| Pears, Comice | 150 |
| Pears, Conference | 170 |
| Pears, Nashi | 150 |
| Pears, William | 150 |
| Physalis | 60 |
| Pineapple | 80 |
| Pineapple, canned in juice | 40 |
| Pineapple, canned in syrup | 40 |
| Plums, average, stewed with sugar | 133 |
| Plums, average, stewed without sugar | 70 |
| Plums, canned in syrup | 80 |
| Plums, Victoria | 55 |
| Plums, yellow | 55 |
| Pomegranate | 55 |
| Pomelo | 80 |
| Prickly pears | 60 |
| Prunes, canned in juice | 24 |

Unless otherwise stated, fruits are prepared but uncooked.

| ENERGY kcal | ENERGY kJ | FAT g | SATURATED FAT g | PROTEIN g | CARBOHYDRATE g | FIBRE g |
|---|---|---|---|---|---|---|
| 66 | 281 | Trace | Trace | 1 | 17 | 0.3 |
| 86 | 368 | 1 | 0.2 | 1 | 21 | 3.9 |
| 81 | 347 | Trace | Trace | 0 | 21 | 0.7 |
| 44 | 184 | Trace | Trace | 0 | 10 | 1 |
| 29 | 122 | Trace | Trace | 1 | 6 | 1.5 |
| 36 | 153 | Trace | Trace | 1 | 8 | 0.6 |
| 56 | 238 | Trace | Trace | 1 | 13 | 1.2 |
| 12 | 49 | Trace | Trace | 0 | 3 | 0.2 |
| 60 | 257 | Trace | Trace | 2 | 14 | 1.8 |
| 59 | 253 | Trace | Trace | 2 | 14 | 2.7 |
| 50 | 214 | Trace | Trace | 1 | 12 | 3.1 |
| 22 | 91 | 1 | 0.1 | 2 | 3 | 2 |
| 36 | 156 | Trace | Trace | 1 | 8 | 1.7 |
| 47 | 198 | Trace | Trace | 1 | 12 | 1 |
| 66 | 280 | Trace | Trace | 1 | 17 | 1.1 |
| 45 | 190 | Trace | Trace | 0 | 11 | 1.9 |
| 68 | 290 | Trace | Trace | 0 | 18 | 1.5 |
| 50 | 212 | Trace | Trace | 0 | 13 | 3 |
| 90 | 386 | 1 | Trace | 1 | 22 | 4.1 |
| 44 | 183 | Trace | Trace | 0 | 11 | 2.3 |
| 51 | 215 | Trace | Trace | 1 | 12 | 3.3 |
| 32 | 131 | Trace | Trace | 1 | 7 | 1 |
| 33 | 141 | Trace | Trace | 0 | 8 | 1 |
| 19 | 80 | Trace | Trace | 0 | 5 | 0.2 |
| 26 | 109 | Trace | Trace | 0 | 7 | 0.3 |
| 105 | 446 | Trace | Trace | 1 | 27 | 1.7 |
| 21 | 90 | Trace | Trace | 0 | 5 | 0.9 |
| 47 | 202 | Trace | Trace | 0 | 12 | 0.6 |
| 21 | 92 | Trace | Trace | 0 | 5 | 1 |
| 14 | 59 | Trace | Trace | 0 | 3 | 0.6 |
| 28 | 120 | Trace | Trace | 1 | 6 | 1.9 |
| 24 | 101 | Trace | Trace | 0 | 5 | 0.8 |
| 29 | 124 | 1 | 0.1 | 0 | 7 | 2.2 |
| 19 | 80 | Trace | Trace | 0 | 5 | 0.6 |

| FRUITS | AVERAGE PORTION g |
|---|---|
| Prunes, canned in syrup | 24 |
| Prunes, dried | 66 |
| Prunes, stewed with sugar | 24 |
| Prunes, stewed without sugar | 24 |
| Quinces | 90 |
| Raisins | 30 |
| Rambutan | 80 |
| Raspberries | 60 |
| Raspberries, canned in syrup | 90 |
| Raspberries, stewed with sugar | 90 |
| Raspberries, stewed without sugar | 90 |
| Redcurrants | 2 |
| Redcurrants, stewed with sugar | 140 |
| Redcurrants, stewed without sugar | 140 |
| Rhubarb, canned in syrup | 140 |
| Rhubarb, stewed with sugar | 140 |
| Rhubarb, stewed without sugar | 140 |
| Satsumas | 70 |
| Sharon fruit | 110 |
| Starfruit | 120 |
| Strawberries | 100 |
| Sugar apples | 60 |
| Sultanas | 18 |
| Tangerines | 70 |
| Watermelon | 200 |

Unless otherwise stated, fruits are prepared but uncooked.

| ENERGY kcal | ENERGY kJ | FAT g | SATURATED FAT g | PROTEIN g | CARBOHYDRATE g | FIBRE g |
|---|---|---|---|---|---|---|
| 22 | 93 | Trace | Trace | 0 | 6 | 0.7 |
| 93 | 397 | Trace | Trace | 2 | 22 | 3.8 |
| 25 | 105 | Trace | Trace | 0 | 6 | 0.7 |
| 19 | 83 | Trace | 0 | 0 | 5 | 0.8 |
| 23 | 99 | Trace | Trace | 0 | 6 | 1.7 |
| 82 | 348 | Trace | Trace | 1 | 21 | 0.6 |
| 55 | 234 | Trace | Trace | 1 | 13 | 0.5 |
| 15 | 65 | 1 | 0.1 | 1 | 3 | 1.5 |
| 79 | 337 | Trace | Trace | 1 | 20 | 1.4 |
| 57 | 244 | 1 | 0.1 | 1 | 14 | 2 |
| 22 | 95 | 1 | 0.1 | 1 | 4 | 2.2 |
| 0 | 2 | Trace | Trace | 0 | 0 | 0.1 |
| 74 | 318 | Trace | Trace | 1 | 19 | 3.8 |
| 24 | 106 | Trace | Trace | 1 | 5 | 4.1 |
| 43 | 182 | Trace | Trace | 1 | 11 | 1.1 |
| 67 | 284 | Trace | Trace | 1 | 16 | 1.7 |
| 10 | 42 | Trace | Trace | 1 | 1 | 1.8 |
| 25 | 109 | Trace | Trace | 1 | 6 | 0.9 |
| 80 | 342 | Trace | Trace | 1 | 20 | 1.8 |
| 38 | 163 | 1 | 0.1 | 1 | 9 | 1.6 |
| 27 | 113 | Trace | Trace | 1 | 6 | 1.1 |
| 41 | 178 | Trace | Trace | 1 | 10 | 1.4 |
| 50 | 211 | Trace | Trace | 0 | 12 | 0.4 |
| 25 | 103 | Trace | Trace | 1 | 6 | 0.9 |
| 62 | 266 | 1 | 0.2 | 1 | 14 | 0.2 |
|  |  |  |  |  |  |  |
|  |  |  |  |  |  |  |
|  |  |  |  |  |  |  |

FRUITS

| VEGETABLES | AVERAGE PORTION g |
|---|---|
| Ackee, canned | 80 |
| Alfalfa sprouts | 5 |
| Artichoke, globe, heart | 40 |
| Artichoke, Jerusalem | 56 |
| Asparagus | 125 |
| Aubergine, fried | 130 |
| Bamboo shoots, canned | 50 |
| **Beans** | |
| Aduki, dried, boiled | 60 |
| Baked, canned in tomato sauce | 135 |
| Baked, canned in tomato sauce, reduced sugar and salt | 135 |
| Baked, canned in tomato sauce, with burgers | 225 |
| Baked, canned in tomato sauce, with pork sausages | 225 |
| Balor, canned | 135 |
| Barbecue, canned in sauce | 135 |
| Blackeye, dried, boiled | 60 |
| Broad | 120 |
| Broad, canned | 120 |
| Broad, frozen | 120 |
| Butter, canned | 120 |
| Butter, dried, boiled | 60 |
| Chickpeas, canned | 70 |
| Chickpeas, split, dried, boiled | 70 |
| Chickpeas, whole, dried, boiled | 70 |
| Chilli, canned | 135 |
| French | 90 |
| French, canned | 90 |
| French, frozen | 90 |
| Green | 90 |
| Green, canned | 90 |
| Green, frozen | 90 |

Unless otherwise stated, vegetables are described as they would normally be eaten.

| ENERGY kcal | ENERGY kJ | FAT g | SATURATED FAT g | PROTEIN g | CARBOHYDRATE g | FIBRE g |
|---|---|---|---|---|---|---|
| 121 | 500 | 12 | Trace | 2 | 1 | 1.4 |
| 1 | 5 | Trace | Trace | 0 | 0 | 0.1 |
| 7 | 31 | 0 | 0 | 1 | 1 | 2 |
| 23 | 116 | Trace | Trace | 1 | 6 | 2 |
| 33 | 138 | 1 | 0.1 | 4 | 2 | 1.7 |
| 393 | 1620 | 41 | 5.3 | 2 | 4 | 3 |
| 6 | 23 | 1 | 0.1 | 1 | 0 | 0.9 |
| | | | | | | |
| 74 | 315 | Trace | Trace | 6 | 14 | 3.3 |
| 109 | 466 | 1 | 0.1 | 6 | 20 | 4.7 |
| | | | | | | |
| 99 | 420 | 1 | 0.1 | 7 | 17 | 5.1 |
| | | | | | | |
| 214 | 900 | 7 | 0.1 | 15 | 25 | 6.8 |
| | | | | | | |
| 239 | 1001 | 10 | 0.1 | 14 | 25 | 6.3 |
| 26 | 112 | Trace | Trace | 3 | 4 | 3.6 |
| 104 | 444 | 1 | 0.1 | 7 | 19 | 4.7 |
| 70 | 296 | 1 | 0.1 | 5 | 12 | 2.1 |
| 58 | 245 | 1 | 0.1 | 6 | 7 | 6.5 |
| 104 | 444 | 1 | 0.1 | 10 | 15 | 6.2 |
| 97 | 413 | 1 | 0.1 | 9 | 14 | 7.8 |
| 92 | 392 | 1 | 0.1 | 7 | 16 | 5.5 |
| 62 | 262 | 1 | 0.1 | 4 | 11 | 3.1 |
| 81 | 341 | 2 | 0.2 | 5 | 11 | 2.9 |
| 80 | 339 | 1 | 0.1 | 5 | 12 | 3 |
| 85 | 358 | 1 | 0.1 | 6 | 13 | 3 |
| 95 | 513 | 1 | 0.1 | 7 | 16 | 5.3 |
| 20 | 83 | 1 | 0.1 | 2 | 3 | 2.2 |
| 20 | 86 | Trace | Trace | 1 | 4 | 2.3 |
| 23 | 97 | Trace | Trace | 2 | 4 | 3.7 |
| 20 | 83 | 1 | 0.1 | 2 | 3 | 2.2 |
| 20 | 86 | Trace | Trace | 1 | 4 | 2.3 |
| 23 | 97 | Trace | Trace | 2 | 4 | 3.7 |

VEGETABLES
& SALADS 17

| VEGETABLES | AVERAGE PORTION g |
|---|---|
| Haricot, dried, boiled | 60 |
| Lilva, canned | 80 |
| Mung, dahl, dried, boiled | 60 |
| Mung, whole, dried, boiled | 60 |
| Papri, canned | 60 |
| Pigeon peas, dahl, dried | 60 |
| Pinto, dried, boiled | 60 |
| Pinto, refried | 60 |
| Red kidney, canned | 60 |
| Red kidney, dried, boiled | 60 |
| Runner | 90 |
| Soya, dried, boiled | 60 |
| Beansprouts, mung | 80 |
| Beansprouts, mung, canned | 80 |
| Beansprouts, mung, stir-fried | 80 |
| Beetroot | 40 |
| Beetroot, pickled | 35 |
| Breadfruit, canned | 40 |
| Broccoli, green | 85 |
| Broccoli, purple sprouting | 85 |
| Brussels sprouts | 90 |
| Cabbage, Chinese | 40 |
| Cabbage, red | 90 |
| Cabbage, red, raw | 90 |
| Cabbage, Savoy | 95 |
| Cabbage, white | 95 |
| Cabbage, white, raw | 90 |
| Carrots, canned | 60 |
| Carrots, old | 60 |
| Carrots, old, raw | 80 |
| Carrots, young | 60 |
| Carrots, young, raw | 60 |
| Cassava, baked | 100 |
| Cauliflower | 90 |

Unless otherwise stated, vegetables are described as they would normally be eaten.

| ENERGY kcal | ENERGY kJ | FAT g | SATURATED FAT g | PROTEIN g | CARBOHYDRATE g | FIBRE g |
|---|---|---|---|---|---|---|
| 57 | 244 | 1 | 0.1 | 4 | 10 | 3.7 |
| 54 | 232 | 1 | 0.1 | 5 | 8 | 0.5 |
| 55 | 235 | 1 | 0.1 | 5 | 9 | 1.8 |
| 55 | 233 | 1 | 0.1 | 5 | 9 | 1.8 |
| 16 | 66 | 1 | 0.1 | 2 | 2 | 0.4 |
| 71 | 298 | 1 | 0.1 | 5 | 13 | 4 |
| 82 | 350 | 1 | 0.1 | 5 | 14 | 2.8 |
| 64 | 268 | 1 | 0.1 | 4 | 9 | 3.2 |
| 60 | 254 | 1 | 0.1 | 4 | 11 | 3.7 |
| 62 | 264 | 1 | 0.1 | 5 | 10 | 4 |
| 16 | 68 | 1 | 0.1 | 1 | 2 | 1.7 |
| 85 | 354 | 4 | 0.5 | 8 | 3 | 3.7 |
| 25 | 105 | 1 | 0.1 | 2 | 3 | 1.2 |
| 8 | 35 | Trace | Trace | 1 | 1 | 0.6 |
| 58 | 238 | 5 | 0.4 | 2 | 2 | 0.7 |
| 18 | 78 | Trace | Trace | 1 | 4 | 0.8 |
| 10 | 41 | Trace | Trace | 0 | 2 | 0.6 |
| 26 | 112 | Trace | Trace | 0 | 7 | 0.7 |
| 20 | 85 | 1 | 0.2 | 3 | 1 | 2 |
| 16 | 68 | 1 | 0.1 | 2 | 1 | 2 |
| 32 | 138 | 1 | 0.3 | 3 | 3 | 2.8 |
| 5 | 20 | Trace | Trace | 0 | 1 | 0.5 |
| 14 | 55 | Trace | Trace | 1 | 2 | 1.8 |
| 19 | 80 | Trace | Trace | 1 | 3 | 2.3 |
| 16 | 67 | 1 | 0.1 | 1 | 2 | 1.9 |
| 13 | 57 | Trace | Trace | 1 | 2 | 1.4 |
| 24 | 102 | Trace | Trace | 1 | 5 | 1.9 |
| 12 | 52 | 1 | 0.1 | 0 | 3 | 1.1 |
| 14 | 60 | 1 | 0.1 | 0 | 3 | 1.5 |
| 28 | 117 | 1 | 0.1 | 0 | 6 | 1.9 |
| 13 | 56 | 1 | 0.1 | 0 | 3 | 1.4 |
| 18 | 75 | 1 | 0.1 | 0 | 4 | 1.4 |
| 155 | 661 | 1 | 0.1 | 1 | 40 | 1.7 |
| 25 | 105 | 1 | 0.2 | 3 | 2 | 1.4 |

VEGETABLES & SALADS

| VEGETABLES | AVERAGE PORTION g |
|---|---|
| Cauliflower, raw | 90 |
| Celeriac | 30 |
| Celeriac, raw | 30 |
| Celery | 30 |
| Chard, Swiss | 90 |
| Chicory, raw | 28 |
| Chilli peppers, capsicum red | 10 |
| Chinese leaf | 40 |
| Corn, on the cob | 200 |
| Courgettes | 90 |
| Courgettes, fried | 90 |
| Cress | 5 |
| Cucumber | 23 |
| Curly kale | 95 |
| Endive | 30 |
| Fennel, Florence | 40 |
| Garlic, raw | 3 |
| Gourd, karela, canned | 30 |
| Jackfruit, canned | 60 |
| Kohlrabi | 60 |
| Kohlrabi, cooked | 90 |
| Leeks | 75 |
| Lentils, canned in tomato sauce | 80 |
| Lentils, green or brown, whole, dried | 80 |
| Lentils, red, split, dried, boiled | 80 |
| Lettuce, Cos | 80 |
| Lettuce, Iceberg | 80 |
| Lettuce, Webbs Wonder | 80 |
| Marrow | 65 |
| Mixed vegetables, frozen | 90 |
| **Mushrooms** | |
| Shiitake, steamed | 40 |
| Straw, canned | 40 |
| White, fried | 44 |

Unless otherwise stated, vegetables are described as they would normally be eaten.

| ENERGY kcal | ENERGY kJ | FAT g | SATURATED FAT g | PROTEIN g | CARBOHYDRATE g | FIBRE g |
|---|---|---|---|---|---|---|
| 31 | 128 | 1 | 0.2 | 3 | 3 | 1.6 |
| 5 | 19 | Trace | Trace | 0 | 1 | 1 |
| 5 | 22 | Trace | Trace | 0 | 1 | 1.1 |
| 2 | 10 | Trace | Trace | 2 | 0 | 0.3 |
| 18 | 76 | Trace | Trace | 2 | 3 | 1.8 |
| 3 | 13 | 1 | 0.1 | 0 | 1 | 0.3 |
| 3 | 11 | Trace | Trace | 0 | 0 | 0.7 |
| 5 | 20 | Trace | Trace | 0 | 1 | 0.5 |
| 132 | 560 | 3 | 0.4 | 5 | 23 | 2.6 |
| 17 | 73 | 1 | 0.1 | 2 | 2 | 1.1 |
| 57 | 239 | 4 | 0.5 | 2 | 2 | 1.1 |
| 1 | 3 | Trace | Trace | 0 | 0 | 0.1 |
| 2 | 9 | Trace | Trace | 0 | 0 | 0.1 |
| 23 | 95 | 1 | 0.2 | 2 | 1 | 2.7 |
| 4 | 16 | 0 | 0 | 1 | 0 | 0.6 |
| 5 | 20 | Trace | Trace | 0 | 1 | 1 |
| 3 | 12 | 0 | 0 | 0 | 0 | 0.1 |
| 3 | 11 | Trace | Trace | 0 | 0 | 0.7 |
| 62 | 264 | Trace | Trace | 0 | 16 | 0.9 |
| 14 | 57 | Trace | Trace | 1 | 2 | 1.3 |
| 16 | 69 | Trace | Trace | 1 | 3 | 1.7 |
| 16 | 65 | 1 | 0.1 | 1 | 2 | 1.3 |
| 44 | 189 | Trace | Trace | 4 | 7 | 1.4 |
| 84 | 357 | 1 | 0.1 | 7 | 14 | 3 |
| 80 | 339 | Trace | Trace | 6 | 14 | 1.5 |
| 13 | 52 | 1 | 0.1 | 1 | 1 | 1 |
| 10 | 42 | Trace | Trace | 1 | 2 | 0.5 |
| 10 | 44 | Trace | Trace | 1 | 2 | 0.6 |
| 6 | 25 | Trace | Trace | 0 | 1 | 0.4 |
| 38 | 162 | Trace | Trace | 3 | 6 | 2.9 |
| 22 | 93 | Trace | 0 | 1 | 5 | 0.8 |
| 6 | 25 | Trace | Trace | 1 | 0 | 1 |
| 69 | 284 | 7 | 0.9 | 1 | 0 | 0.7 |

## VEGETABLES

| | AVERAGE PORTION g |
|---|---|
| White, raw | 40 |
| Okra | 30 |
| Onions | 150 |
| Onions, fried | 40 |
| Parsnips | 65 |
| Parsnips, roasted without oil | 90 |
| Peas, canned | 70 |
| Peas, fresh | 70 |
| Peas, frozen | 70 |
| Peas, mangetout, stir-fried | 90 |
| Peas, marrowfat, canned | 80 |
| Peas, mushy, canned | 80 |
| Peas, petit pois, canned | 70 |
| Peas, petit pois, frozen | 70 |
| Peas, sugar-snap | 90 |
| Pease pudding, canned | 80 |
| Peppers, capsicum, green | 160 |
| Peppers, capsicum, red | 160 |
| Peppers, capsicum, yellow | 160 |
| Plantain | 200 |
| Plantain, ripe, fried | 200 |
| **Potatoes and potato products** | |
| Chips, crinkle cut, frozen, fried | 165 |
| Chips, fine cut, frozen, fried | 165 |
| Chips, fried | 165 |
| Chips, shop bought, fried | 165 |
| Chips, straight cut, frozen, fried | 165 |
| Chips, thick cut, frozen, fried | 165 |
| Croquettes, fried | 180 |
| Duchesse | 120 |
| French fries | 110 |
| Microwave chips | 165 |
| Instant mash, made with semi-skimmed milk | 60 |

Unless otherwise stated, vegetables are described as they would normally be eaten.

| ENERGY kcal | ENERGY kJ | FAT g | SATURATED FAT g | PROTEIN g | CARBOHYDRATE g | FIBRE g |
|---|---|---|---|---|---|---|
| 5 | 22 | Trace | 0 | 1 | 0 | 0.4 |
| 8 | 36 | 1 | 0.1 | 1 | 1 | 1.1 |
| 54 | 225 | Trace | Trace | 2 | 12 | 2.1 |
| 66 | 274 | 4 | 0.6 | 1 | 6 | 1.2 |
| 43 | 181 | 1 | 0.1 | 1 | 8 | 3.1 |
| 102 | 427 | 6 | Trace | 1 | 12 | 4.2 |
| 56 | 237 | 1 | 0.1 | 4 | 9 | 3.6 |
| 55 | 230 | 1 | 0.2 | 5 | 7 | 3.2 |
| 48 | 204 | 1 | 0.1 | 4 | 7 | 3.6 |
| 64 | 268 | 4 | 0.4 | 3 | 3 | 2.2 |
| 80 | 329 | 1 | 0.1 | 6 | 14 | 3.3 |
| 65 | 276 | 1 | 0.1 | 5 | 11 | 1.4 |
| 32 | 132 | 1 | 0.1 | 4 | 3 | 3 |
| 34 | 144 | 1 | 0.1 | 4 | 4 | 3.2 |
| 30 | 125 | 1 | 0.1 | 3 | 4 | 1.2 |
| 74 | 316 | 1 | 0.1 | 5 | 13 | 1.4 |
| 24 | 104 | 1 | 0.2 | 1 | 4 | 2.6 |
| 51 | 214 | 1 | 0.2 | 2 | 10 | 2.6 |
| 42 | 181 | Trace | Trace | 2 | 8 | 2.7 |
| 224 | 954 | 1 | 0.2 | 2 | 57 | 2.4 |
| 534 | 2252 | 1 | 2 | 3 | 95 | 4.6 |
| | | | | | | |
| 479 | 2001 | 28 | 5.1 | 6 | 55 | 3.6 |
| 601 | 2515 | 35 | 8.6 | 7 | 68 | 4.5 |
| 312 | 1313 | 11 | 1.5 | 6 | 50 | 3.6 |
| 394 | 1652 | 20 | 2.6 | 5 | 50 | 3.6 |
| 450 | 1889 | 22 | 4.1 | 7 | 59 | 4 |
| 386 | 1622 | 17 | 3.1 | 6 | 56 | 4 |
| 385 | 1607 | 24 | 3.1 | 7 | 39 | 2.3 |
| 148 | 622 | 6 | 3.6 | 4 | 20 | 1.4 |
| 308 | 1291 | 17 | 6.4 | 4 | 37 | 2.3 |
| 365 | 1535 | 17 | 3 | 6 | 53 | 4.8 |
| | | | | | | |
| 42 | 178 | 1 | 0.2 | 1 | 9 | 0.6 |

VEGETABLES
& SALADS

## VEGETABLES

| | AVERAGE PORTION g |
|---|---|
| Instant mash, made with water | 60 |
| Instant mash, made with whole milk | 60 |
| New, canned | 165 |
| New, chipped, fried | 165 |
| New, in skins, boiled | 175 |
| Old, baked | 180 |
| Old, boiled | 175 |
| Old, mashed with butter | 120 |
| Old, mashed with polyunsaturated fat spread | 120 |
| Old, roast | 130 |
| Oven chips, frozen | 165 |
| Oven chips, thick cut, frozen | 165 |
| Waffles, frozen | 90 |
| Wedges, baked | 180 |
| Pumpkin | 60 |
| Raddiccio, raw | 30 |
| Radishes, red, raw | 48 |
| Salad onions | 10 |
| Sauerkraut | 30 |
| Spinach | 90 |
| Spinach, cooked | 90 |
| Split peas, dried, boiled | 90 |
| Spring greens, boiled | 95 |
| Spring onions | 10 |
| Squash, acorn, baked | 65 |
| Squash, butternut, baked | 65 |
| Squash, spaghetti, baked | 65 |
| Swede | 60 |
| Sweet potato | 130 |
| Sweet potato, baked | 130 |
| Sweetcorn, baby, canned | 60 |
| Sweetcorn kernels, canned, reheated | 85 |
| Tomatoes | 85 |

Unless otherwise stated, vegetables are described as they would normally be eaten.

| ENERGY kcal | ENERGY kJ | FAT g | SATURATED FAT g | PROTEIN g | CARBOHYDRATE g | FIBRE g |
|---|---|---|---|---|---|---|
| 34 | 147 | Trace | Trace | 1 | 8 | 0.6 |
| 46 | 193 | 1 | 0.4 | 1 | 9 | 0.6 |
| 104 | 447 | Trace | Trace | 2 | 25 | 1.3 |
| 376 | 1582 | 16 | 2 | 7 | 55 | 2.8 |
| 116 | 492 | 1 | 0.2 | 2 | 27 | 2.6 |
| 245 | 1046 | Trace | Trace | 7 | 57 | 4.9 |
| 126 | 536 | Trace | Trace | 3 | 30 | 2.1 |
| 125 | 526 | 5 | 3.4 | 2 | 19 | 1.3 |
| | | | | | | |
| 125 | 526 | 5 | 1.1 | 2 | 19 | 1.3 |
| 194 | 819 | 6 | 0.8 | 4 | 34 | 2.3 |
| 267 | 1134 | 7 | 3 | 5 | 49 | 3.3 |
| 259 | 1096 | 7 | 2.8 | 5 | 46 | 3 |
| 180 | 758 | 12 | 1 | 2 | 28 | 2 |
| 245 | 1046 | Trace | Trace | 7 | 57 | 4.9 |
| 8 | 34 | 1 | 0.1 | 0 | 1 | 0.7 |
| 4 | 17 | Trace | Trace | 0 | 1 | 0.5 |
| 6 | 24 | 0 | 0 | 0 | 1 | 0.4 |
| 2 | 10 | 0 | 0 | 0 | 0 | 0.2 |
| 3 | 11 | Trace | Trace | 0 | 0 | 0.7 |
| 23 | 93 | 1 | 0.1 | 3 | 1 | 1.9 |
| 17 | 71 | 1 | 0.1 | 2 | 1 | 1.9 |
| 113 | 484 | 1 | 0.2 | 7 | 20 | 2.4 |
| 19 | 78 | 1 | 0.1 | 2 | 2 | 2.5 |
| 2 | 10 | 0 | 0 | 0 | 0 | 0.2 |
| 36 | 152 | Trace | Trace | 1 | 8 | 2.1 |
| 21 | 89 | Trace | Trace | 1 | 5 | 0.9 |
| 15 | 62 | Trace | 0.1 | 0 | 3 | 1.4 |
| 7 | 28 | Trace | Trace | 0 | 1 | 0.4 |
| 109 | 465 | 1 | 0.1 | 1 | 27 | 3 |
| 150 | 634 | 1 | 0.3 | 2 | 36 | 4.3 |
| 14 | 58 | Trace | Trace | 2 | 1 | 0.9 |
| 104 | 441 | 1 | 0.2 | 2 | 23 | 1.2 |
| 14 | 62 | 1 | 0.1 | 1 | 3 | 0.9 |

VEGETABLES
& SALADS 2

## VEGETABLES

| | AVERAGE PORTION g |
|---|---|
| Tomatoes, canned, not drained | 200 |
| Tomatoes, cherry | 90 |
| Tomatoes, fried | 85 |
| Tomatoes, grilled | 85 |
| Turnips | 60 |
| Water chestnuts, canned | 28 |
| Watercress | 20 |
| Yam | 130 |
| Yam, baked | 130 |
| Yam, steamed | 130 |

## PREPARED SALADS

| | |
|---|---|
| Baby leaf salad | 50 |
| Bean salad | 200 |
| Beetroot salad | 100 |
| Carrot and nut salad with French dressing | 95 |
| Coleslaw, with mayonnaise | 100 |
| Coleslaw, with reduced-calorie dressing | 100 |
| Coleslaw, with vinaigrette | 100 |
| Florida salad | 95 |
| Greek salad | 95 |
| Green salad | 95 |
| Herb salad | 50 |
| Pasta salad | 95 |
| Pasta salad, wholemeal | 95 |
| Potato salad, with mayonnaise | 85 |
| Potato salad, with reduced-calorie mayonnaise | 85 |
| Rice salad | 90 |
| Rice salad, brown | 95 |
| Rocket salad | 25 |
| Tabbouleh | 100 |

Unless otherwise stated, vegetables are described as they would normally be eaten.

| ENERGY kcal | ENERGY kJ | FAT g | SATURATED FAT g | PROTEIN g | CARBOHYDRATE g | FIBRE g |
|---|---|---|---|---|---|---|
| 32 | 138 | Trace | Trace | 2 | 6 | 1.4 |
| 16 | 68 | 1 | 0.1 | 1 | 3 | 0.9 |
| 77 | 320 | 7 | 0.9 | 1 | 4 | 1.1 |
| 42 | 179 | 1 | 0.3 | 2 | 8 | 2.5 |
| 7 | 31 | 1 | Trace | 0 | 1 | 1.1 |
| 9 | 37 | Trace | Trace | 0 | 3 | 2 |
| 4 | 19 | 1 | 0.1 | 1 | 0 | 0.3 |
| 173 | 738 | 1 | 0.1 | 2 | 43 | 1.8 |
| 199 | 846 | 1 | 0.1 | 3 | 49 | 2.2 |
| 148 | 634 | 1 | 0.1 | 2 | 37 | 1.7 |
| | | | | | | |
| 9 | 40 | Trace | Trace | Trace | 2 | 0.7 |
| 294 | 1236 | 19 | 2 | 8 | 26 | 6 |
| 100 | 417 | 7 | 0.7 | 2 | 8 | 1.7 |
| 207 | 858 | 17 | 1.6 | 2 | 13 | 2.3 |
| 258 | 939 | 26 | 3.9 | 1 | 4 | 1.4 |
| 67 | 280 | 5 | 0.5 | 1 | 6 | 1.4 |
| 87 | 364 | 4 | 0.5 | 1 | 12 | 1.7 |
| 213 | 790 | 19 | 2.9 | 1 | 9 | 1 |
| 124 | 513 | 12 | 3.1 | 3 | 2 | 0.8 |
| 11 | 48 | 0 | Trace | 1 | 2 | 1 |
| 9 | 40 | Trace | Trace | Trace | Trace | 0.7 |
| 121 | 473 | 7 | 1 | 2 | 13 | 1.5 |
| 124 | 493 | 7 | 1 | 3 | 13 | 2.8 |
| 203 | 757 | 18 | 2.6 | 1 | 10 | 0.8 |
| 82 | 349 | 3 | 0.3 | 1 | 13 | 0.7 |
| 149 | 628 | 7 | 1 | 3 | 21 | 0.6 |
| 159 | 668 | 7 | 1 | 3 | 23 | 1 |
| 3 | 12 | Trace | Trace | Trace | Trace | 0.2 |
| 119 | 496 | 5 | 0.4 | 3 | 17 | 1 |

VEGETABLES
& SALADS

## PREPARED SALADS

| | AVERAGE PORTION g |
|---|---|
| Tomato and onion salad | 90 |
| Waldorf salad | 90 |

## VEGETABLE DISHES, HOMEMADE

| | |
|---|---|
| Bean loaf | 90 |
| Bhaji, aubergine, pea, potato and cauliflower | 70 |
| Bhaji, potato and cauliflower, fried | 70 |
| Bhaji, potato and onion | 70 |
| Broccoli in cheese sauce, made with semi-skimmed milk | 190 |
| Broccoli in cheese sauce, made with whole milk | 190 |
| Bubble and squeak, fried | 140 |
| Cannelloni, spinach | 340 |
| Cannelloni, vegetable | 340 |
| Casserole, vegetable | 220 |
| Cauliflower cheese, made with semi-skimmed milk | 200 |
| Cauliflower cheese, made with whole milk | 200 |
| Cauliflower in white sauce, made with skimmed milk | 200 |
| Cauliflower in white sauce, made with whole milk | 200 |
| Chilli, bean and lentil | 290 |
| Chilli, vegetable | 220 |
| Curry, chickpea | 210 |
| Curry, potato and pea | 290 |
| Curry, vegetable | 200 |
| Dahl, mung bean, dried, boiled | 60 |
| Dahl, pigeon peas, dried, boiled | 60 |
| Falafel, fried | 100 |

Unless otherwise stated, vegetables are described as they would normally be eaten.

| ENERGY kcal | ENERGY kJ | FAT g | SATURATED FAT g | PROTEIN g | CARBOHYDRATE g | FIBRE g |
|---|---|---|---|---|---|---|
| 65 | 272 | 5 | 0.6 | 1 | 4 | 0.9 |
| 174 | 662 | 16 | 2.1 | 1 | 7 | 1.2 |
| 134 | 564 | 7 | 0.7 | 6 | 14 | 3.9 |
| 49 | 209 | 2 | 0.2 | 2 | 7 | 2 |
| 214 | 888 | 15 | 1.8 | 5 | 14 | 2.7 |
| 112 | 468 | 7 | 4.6 | 1 | 12 | 1.1 |
| 211 | 880 | 14 | 7.2 | 12 | 9 | 2.9 |
| 224 | 939 | 16 | 8.2 | 12 | 9 | 2.9 |
| 174 | 727 | 13 | 1.4 | 2 | 14 | 2.1 |
| 449 | 1880 | 26 | 7.8 | 15 | 43 | 2.7 |
| 493 | 2067 | 31 | 11.6 | 15 | 43 | 2.4 |
| 114 | 486 | 1 | 0.2 | 5 | 23 | 4.6 |
| 200 | 840 | 13 | 6 | 12 | 10 | 2.6 |
| 210 | 880 | 14 | 6.6 | 12 | 10 | 2.6 |
| 122 | 512 | 6 | 2.2 | 7 | 10 | 2.2 |
| 136 | 568 | 8 | 3.2 | 7 | 10 | 2.2 |
| 264 | 1111 | 8 | 0.9 | 15 | 38 | 10.4 |
| 125 | 532 | 1 | 0.2 | 7 | 24 | 5.7 |
| 227 | 956 | 8 | 0.8 | 13 | 30 | 6.9 |
| 267 | 1122 | 11 | 1.2 | 8 | 38 | 7 |
| 176 | 736 | 12 | 1.2 | 5 | 14 | 5 |
| 55 | 235 | 1 | 0.1 | 5 | 9 | 1.8 |
| 71 | 298 | 1 | 0.1 | 5 | 13 | 4 |
| 179 | 750 | 11 | 1.1 | 6 | 16 | 3.4 |

## VEGETABLE DISHES, HOMEMADE

| | AVERAGE PORTION g |
|---|---|
| Lasagne, spinach | 420 |
| Lasagne, spinach, wholemeal | 420 |
| Lasagne, vegetable | 420 |
| Lasagne, vegetable, wholemeal | 420 |
| Lentil and nut roast | 100 |
| Lentil pie | 100 |
| Lentil roast | 100 |
| Moussaka, vegetable | 330 |
| Pakora, potato and cauliflower, fried | 70 |
| Pasty, vegetable | 155 |
| Pasty, vegetable, wholemeal | 155 |
| Peppers, stuffed with rice | 175 |
| Peppers, stuffed with vegetables, cheese topping | 175 |
| Pilau, mushroom | 180 |
| Pilau, vegetable | 180 |
| Quiche, broccoli | 140 |
| Quiche, broccoli, wholemeal | 140 |
| Quiche, cauliflower cheese | 140 |
| Quiche, cauliflower cheese, wholemeal | 140 |
| Quiche, cheese and egg | 140 |
| Quiche, cheese and egg, wholemeal | 140 |
| Quiche, cheese and mushroom | 140 |
| Quiche, cheese and mushroom, wholemeal | 140 |
| Quiche, cheese, onion and potato | 140 |
| Quiche, cheese, onion and potato, wholemeal | 140 |
| Quiche, mushroom | 140 |
| Quiche, mushroom, wholemeal | 140 |
| Quiche, spinach | 140 |
| Quiche, spinach, wholemeal | 140 |
| Quiche, vegetable | 140 |
| Quiche, vegetable, wholemeal | 140 |

Unless otherwise stated, vegetables are described as they would normally be eaten.

| ENERGY kcal | ENERGY kJ | FAT g | SATURATED FAT g | PROTEIN g | CARBOHYDRATE g | FIBRE g |
|---|---|---|---|---|---|---|
| 365 | 1541 | 13 | 5.5 | 15 | 53 | 4.6 |
| 391 | 1659 | 13 | 5.5 | 18 | 55 | 9.7 |
| 428 | 1810 | 18 | 9.2 | 17 | 52 | 4.2 |
| 445 | 1877 | 19 | 9.2 | 20 | 52 | 8.8 |
| 222 | 929 | 12 | 1.8 | 11 | 19 | 3.8 |
| 156 | 659 | 4 | 0.5 | 7 | 24 | 3.8 |
| 139 | 588 | 3 | 0.4 | 8 | 22 | 3.4 |
| 452 | 1888 | 31 | 9.2 | 15 | 30 | 4 |
| 214 | 888 | 15 | 1.8 | 5 | 14 | 2.7 |
| 425 | 1783 | 23 | 5.7 | 6 | 52 | 2.9 |
| 406 | 1702 | 24 | 5.7 | 8 | 43 | 6.4 |
| 149 | 630 | 4 | 0.7 | 3 | 27 | 2.3 |
| | | | | | | |
| 194 | 810 | 12 | 3.5 | 6 | 17 | 2.6 |
| 248 | 1048 | 8 | 4.5 | 4 | 43 | 0.7 |
| 248 | 1053 | 8 | 4.3 | 5 | 43 | 1 |
| 349 | 1455 | 21 | 8.3 | 12 | 30 | 1.7 |
| 337 | 1408 | 21 | 8.3 | 13 | 25 | 3.8 |
| 277 | 1156 | 18 | 7.1 | 7 | 24 | 1.5 |
| 269 | 1121 | 18 | 7.1 | 8 | 20 | 3.1 |
| 440 | 1834 | 31 | 14.4 | 18 | 24 | 0.8 |
| 431 | 1796 | 31 | 14.6 | 18 | 20 | 2.7 |
| 396 | 1655 | 26 | 10.8 | 15 | 26 | 1.3 |
| | | | | | | |
| 388 | 1616 | 27 | 10.8 | 16 | 22 | 3.1 |
| 480 | 2005 | 33 | 16 | 18 | 28 | 1.4 |
| | | | | | | |
| 472 | 1966 | 34 | 16.1 | 19 | 25 | 3.1 |
| 398 | 1659 | 27 | 12.2 | 14 | 26 | 1.3 |
| 388 | 1618 | 28 | 12.2 | 15 | 21 | 3.1 |
| 287 | 1203 | 18 | 5.6 | 14 | 18 | 2 |
| 281 | 1176 | 18 | 5.6 | 15 | 16 | 3.2 |
| 295 | 1238 | 18 | 6 | 7 | 28 | 2.1 |
| 286 | 1197 | 18 | 6 | 8 | 24 | 3.9 |

VEGETABLES & SALADS **31**

| VEGETABLE DISHES, HOMEMADE | AVERAGE PORTION g |
| --- | --- |
| Refried beans | 90 |
| Rice and blackeye beans | 200 |
| Rice and blackeye beans, brown rice | 200 |
| Risotto, vegetable | 290 |
| Risotto, vegetable, brown rice | 290 |
| Rissoles, chickpea, fried | 100 |
| Rissoles, lentil, fried | 100 |
| Vegetable bake | 260 |
| Vine leaves, stuffed with rice | 80 |

## VEGETARIAN PRODUCTS AND DISHES

| | |
| --- | --- |
| Beanburger, aduki, fried | 90 |
| Beanburger, butter bean, fried | 90 |
| Beanburger, red kidney bean, fried | 90 |
| Beanburger, soya, fried | 90 |
| Quorn™, myco-protein | 90 |
| Tempeh | 60 |
| Tofu, fried | 80 |
| Tofu, steamed | 80 |
| Tofu, steamed, fried | 80 |
| Tofu burger, baked | 9 |
| Vegebanger mix, made with water and egg, fried | 56 |
| Vegebanger mix, made with water, fried | 56 |
| Vegeburger, fried | 56 |
| Vegeburger, grilled | 56 |
| Vegeburger mix, made with water and egg, fried | 56 |
| Vegeburger mix, made with water and egg, grilled | 56 |
| Vegeburger mix, made with water, fried | 56 |
| Vegeburger mix, made with water, grilled | 56 |

Unless otherwise stated, vegetables are described as they would normally be eaten.

| ENERGY kcal | ENERGY kJ | FAT g | SATURATED FAT g | PROTEIN g | CARBOHYDRATE g | FIBRE g |
|---|---|---|---|---|---|---|
| 211 | 885 | 12 | 2.7 | 9 | 18 | 6.3 |
| 366 | 1556 | 7 | 3 | 12 | 68 | 2.8 |
| 350 | 1488 | 7 | 3 | 11 | 66 | 3.6 |
| 426 | 1798 | 19 | 2.9 | 12 | 56 | 6.4 |
| 415 | 1749 | 19 | 2.6 | 12 | 54 | 7 |
| 243 | 1016 | 17 | 1.9 | 8 | 16 | 4.1 |
| 211 | 886 | 11 | 1.3 | 9 | 22 | 3.6 |
| 330 | 1383 | 18 | 7.8 | 11 | 32 | 2.9 |
| 210 | 875 | 14 | 2.1 | 2 | 19 | 1.0 |
| | | | | | | |
| 165 | 695 | 6 | 0.9 | 7 | 21 | 3.9 |
| 172 | 722 | 10 | 1.1 | 5 | 17 | 3.7 |
| 183 | 768 | 10 | 1.1 | 6 | 20 | 4.4 |
| 174 | 725 | 10 | 1.4 | 10 | 12 | 4.2 |
| 77 | 326 | 3 | Trace | 11 | 2 | 4.3 |
| 100 | 418 | 4 | 2 | 12 | 4 | 2.6 |
| 242 | 1011 | 20 | 2.3 | 17 | 3 | 1 |
| 58 | 243 | 3 | 0.4 | 6 | 1 | 1 |
| 209 | 869 | 14 | 2.3 | 19 | 2 | 1 |
| 11 | 45 | 0 | 0.1 | 1 | 1 | 0.2 |
| | | | | | | |
| 157 | 659 | 10 | 2.5 | 10 | 7 | 1.9 |
| 137 | 572 | 9 | 2 | 8 | 7 | 1.8 |
| 137 | 571 | 10 | 1.7 | 9 | 4 | 2 |
| 110 | 460 | 6 | 1.7 | 9 | 4 | 2.4 |
| | | | | | | |
| 122 | 511 | 7 | 1.6 | 8 | 7 | 1.8 |
| | | | | | | |
| 91 | 385 | 4 | 1.2 | 8 | 7 | 1.8 |
| 115 | 482 | 6 | 1.3 | 7 | 8 | 2 |
| | | | | | | |
| 84 | 356 | 3 | 1 | 7 | 8 | 2 |

VEGETABLES
& SALADS 33

| BEEF | AVERAGE PORTION g |
|------|------------------|
| Braising steak, braised | 140 |
| Braising steak, untrimmed, braised | 140 |
| Braising steak, slow cooked | 140 |
| Braising steak, untrimmed, slow cooked | 140 |
| Fillet steak, fried | 172 |
| Fillet steak, untrimmed, fried | 172 |
| Fillet steak, grilled | 168 |
| Fillet steak, untrimmed, grilled | 168 |
| Flank, pot roasted | 140 |
| Flank, untrimmed, pot roasted | 140 |
| Fore rib, roasted | 90 |
| Fore rib, untrimmed, roasted | 90 |
| Mince, extra lean, stewed | 140 |
| Mince, microwaved | 140 |
| Mince, stewed | 140 |
| Rib roast, roasted | 90 |
| Rib roast, untrimmed, roasted | 90 |
| Rump steak, grilled | 163 |
| Rump steak, untrimmed, grilled | 163 |
| Rump steak, fried | 166 |
| Rump steak, untrimmed, fried | 166 |
| Rump steak strips, stir-fried | 103 |
| Rump steak strips, untrimmed, stir-fried | 103 |
| Silverside, pot roasted | 140 |
| Silverside, untrimmed, pot roasted | 140 |
| Silverside, salted, boiled | 140 |
| Silverside, untrimmed, salted, boiled | 140 |
| Sirloin joint, roasted | 90 |
| Sirloin joint, untrimmed, roasted | 90 |
| Sirloin steak, fried | 169 |
| Sirloin steak, untrimmed, fried | 169 |
| Sirloin steak, grilled medium rare | 166 |
| Sirloin steak, untrimmed, grilled medium rare | 166 |

Unless otherwise stated, all meat is lean and trimmed, and all chops and cutlets are boned. Steaks are medium-sized. Unless stated otherwise, all dishes are homemade.

| ENERGY kcal | ENERGY kJ | FAT g | SATURATED FAT g | PROTEIN g | CARBOHYDRATE g | FIBRE g |
|---|---|---|---|---|---|---|
| 315 | 1322 | 14 | 5.7 | 48 | 0 | 0 |
| 344 | 1441 | 18 | 7.4 | 46 | 0 | 0 |
| 276 | 1156 | 11 | 4.8 | 44 | 0 | 0 |
| 304 | 1270 | 16 | 6.7 | 41 | 0 | 0 |
| 316 | 1328 | 14 | 5.8 | 49 | 0 | 0 |
| 330 | 1384 | 15 | 6.7 | 49 | 0 | 0 |
| 316 | 1329 | 13 | 6 | 49 | 0 | 0 |
| 336 | 1410 | 16 | 7.4 | 48 | 0 | 0 |
| 354 | 1483 | 20 | 8 | 45 | 0 | 0 |
| 433 | 1800 | 31 | 12.7 | 38 | 0 | 0 |
| 212 | 889 | 10 | 4.6 | 30 | 0 | 0 |
| 270 | 1125 | 18 | 8.3 | 26 | 0 | 0 |
| 248 | 1039 | 12 | 5.3 | 35 | 0 | 0 |
| 368 | 1534 | 25 | 10.6 | 37 | 0 | 0 |
| 293 | 1218 | 19 | 8.3 | 31 | 0 | 0 |
| 212 | 889 | 10 | 4.6 | 30 | 0 | 0 |
| 270 | 1125 | 18 | 8.3 | 26 | 0 | 0 |
| 287 | 1208 | 9 | 3.9 | 51 | 0 | 0 |
| 331 | 1384 | 15 | 6.5 | 48 | 0 | 0 |
| 304 | 1278 | 11 | 4.2 | 51 | 0 | 0 |
| 378 | 1582 | 21 | 8.1 | 47 | 0 | 0 |
| 214 | 901 | 9 | 3.4 | 33 | 0 | 0 |
| 255 | 1069 | 15 | 5.8 | 31 | 0 | 0 |
| 270 | 1135 | 9 | 3.5 | 48 | 0 | 0 |
| 346 | 1448 | 19 | 7.8 | 43 | 0 | 0 |
| 258 | 1081 | 10 | 3.5 | 43 | 0 | 0 |
| 314 | 1312 | 18 | 6.6 | 39 | 0 | 0 |
| 169 | 712 | 6 | 2.6 | 29 | 0 | 0 |
| 210 | 876 | 11 | 5 | 27 | 0 | 0 |
| 319 | 1340 | 14 | 5.7 | 49 | 0 | 0 |
| 394 | 1646 | 24 | 10.1 | 45 | 0 | 0 |
| 292 | 1223 | 13 | 5.6 | 44 | 0 | 0 |
| 354 | 1474 | 21 | 9.3 | 41 | 0 | 0 |

MEAT &
MEAT DISHES **35**

| BEEF | AVERAGE PORTION g |
|---|---|
| Sirloin steak, grilled rare | 166 |
| Sirloin steak, untrimmed, grilled rare | 166 |
| Sirloin steak, grilled well done | 166 |
| Sirloin steak, untrimmed, grilled well done | 166 |
| Stewing steak, stewed | 140 |
| Stewing steak, untrimmed, stewed | 140 |
| Topside, roasted medium rare | 90 |
| Topside, untrimmed, roasted medium rare | 90 |
| Topside, roasted well done | 90 |
| Topside, untrimmed, roasted well done | 90 |

| LAMB | |
|---|---|
| Best end neck cutlets, grilled | 50 |
| Best end neck cutlets, untrimmed, grilled | 50 |
| Breast, roasted | 90 |
| Breast, untrimmed, roasted | 90 |
| Chump chops, fried | 70 |
| Chump chops, untrimmed, fried | 70 |
| Chump steaks, untrimmed, fried | 90 |
| Kebabs, grilled | 90 |
| Leg, roasted medium | 90 |
| Leg, untrimmed, roasted medium | 90 |
| Leg, roasted well done | 90 |
| Leg, untrimmed, roasted well done | 90 |
| Leg chops, untrimmed, grilled | 70 |
| Leg half fillet, braised | 70 |
| Leg half fillet, untrimmed, braised | 70 |
| Leg half knuckle, pot roasted | 90 |
| Leg half knuckle, untrimmed, pot roasted | 90 |
| Leg joint, roasted | 90 |

Unless otherwise stated, all meat is lean and trimmed, and all chops and
cutlets are boned. Steaks are medium-sized. Unless stated otherwise, all
dishes are homemade.

| ENERGY kcal | ENERGY kJ | FAT g | SATURATED FAT g | PROTEIN g | CARBOHYDRATE g | FIBRE g |
|---|---|---|---|---|---|---|
| 276 | 1157 | 11 | 5 | 44 | 0 | 0 |
| 359 | 1494 | 21 | 9.6 | 42 | 0 | 0 |
| 374 | 1565 | 16 | 7.3 | 56 | 0 | 0 |
| | | | | | | |
| 427 | 1781 | 24 | 10.8 | 53 | 0 | 0 |
| 259 | 1088 | 9 | 3.2 | 45 | 0 | 0 |
| 284 | 1193 | 13 | 5.2 | 41 | 0 | 0 |
| 158 | 662 | 5 | 1.9 | 29 | 0 | 0 |
| | | | | | | |
| 200 | 837 | 10 | 4.3 | 27 | 0 | 0 |
| 182 | 764 | 6 | 2.3 | 33 | 0 | 0 |
| 220 | 918 | 11 | 4.7 | 30 | 0 | 0 |
| | | | | | | |
| | | | | | | |
| 118 | 493 | 7 | 3.3 | 14 | 0 | 0 |
| | | | | | | |
| 171 | 710 | 14 | 6.6 | 12 | 0 | 0 |
| 246 | 1024 | 17 | 7.7 | 24 | 0 | 0 |
| 323 | 1338 | 27 | 12.9 | 20 | 0 | 0 |
| 149 | 624 | 8 | 3.5 | 20 | 0 | 0 |
| 216 | 895 | 16 | 7.6 | 17 | 0 | 0 |
| 255 | 1058 | 18 | 8.5 | 22 | 0 | 0 |
| 259 | 1079 | 17 | 8.1 | 26 | 0 | 0 |
| 183 | 768 | 8 | 3.4 | 27 | 0 | 0 |
| 216 | 904 | 13 | 5.3 | 25 | 0 | 0 |
| 187 | 786 | 8 | 3.3 | 28 | 0 | 0 |
| 218 | 909 | 12 | 5.1 | 27 | 0 | 0 |
| 155 | 648 | 8 | 3.5 | 20 | 0 | 0 |
| 143 | 597 | 7 | 3.2 | 19 | 0 | 0 |
| 179 | 748 | 12 | 5.4 | 18 | 0 | 0 |
| 181 | 760 | 8 | 3.5 | 26 | 0 | 0 |
| 213 | 889 | 12 | 5.4 | 25 | 0 | 0 |
| 189 | 791 | 9 | 3.1 | 28 | 0 | 0 |

MEAT &
MEAT DISHES

| LAMB | AVERAGE PORTION g |
|---|---|
| Leg joint, untrimmed, roasted | 90 |
| Leg steaks, grilled | 90 |
| Leg steaks, untrimmed, grilled | 90 |
| Loin chops, grilled | 70 |
| Loin chops, untrimmed, grilled | 70 |
| Loin chops, roasted | 70 |
| Loin chops, untrimmed, roasted | 70 |
| Loin joint, roasted | 90 |
| Loin joint, untrimmed, roasted | 90 |
| Mince, stewed | 90 |
| Neck fillet, grilled | 90 |
| Neck fillet, untrimmed, grilled | 90 |
| Neck fillet strips, stir-fried | 90 |
| Neck fillet strips, untrimmed, stir-fried | 90 |
| Rack of lamb, roasted | 90 |
| Rack of lamb, untrimmed, roasted | 90 |
| Shoulder half bladeside, pot roasted | 90 |
| Shoulder half bladeside, untrimmed, pot roasted | 90 |
| Shoulder half knuckle, braised | 90 |
| Shoulder half knuckle, untrimmed, braised | 90 |
| Shoulder joint, roasted | 90 |
| Shoulder joint, untrimmed, roasted | 90 |
| Shoulder, roasted | 90 |
| Shoulder, untrimmed, roasted | 90 |
| Stewing lamb, stewed | 260 |
| Stewing lamb, untrimmed, stewed | 260 |

Unless otherwise stated, all meat is lean and trimmed, and all chops and
cutlets are boned. Steaks are medium-sized. Unless stated otherwise, all
dishes are homemade.

| ENERGY kcal | ENERGY kJ | FAT g | SATURATED FAT g | PROTEIN g | CARBOHYDRATE g | FIBRE g |
|---|---|---|---|---|---|---|
| 212 | 887 | 12 | 4.2 | 27 | 0 | 0 |
| 178 | 746 | 8 | 3.2 | 26 | 0 | 0 |
| 208 | 868 | 12 | 5 | 25 | 0 | 0 |
| 149 | 624 | 7 | 3.4 | 20 | 0 | 0 |
| 214 | 888 | 15 | 7.4 | 19 | 0 | 0 |
| 180 | 754 | 9 | 4.3 | 24 | 0 | 0 |
| 251 | 1043 | 19 | 9 | 20 | 0 | 0 |
| 188 | 788 | 10 | 4.4 | 25 | 0 | 0 |
| 273 | 1133 | 20 | 9.5 | 23 | 0 | 0 |
| 187 | 783 | 11 | 5.2 | 22 | 0 | 0 |
| 256 | 1063 | 17 | 7.8 | 25 | 0 | 0 |
| 272 | 1131 | 20 | 9.3 | 24 | 0 | 0 |
| 250 | 1040 | 18 | 7.4 | 22 | 0 | 0 |
| 271 | 1124 | 21 | 8.9 | 21 | 0 | 0 |
| 203 | 848 | 12 | 5.6 | 24 | 0 | 0 |
| 327 | 1355 | 27 | 13.3 | 21 | 0 | 0 |
| 211 | 878 | 13 | 5.8 | 24 | 0 | 0 |
| 292 | 1212 | 23 | 10.8 | 21 | 0 | 0 |
| 191 | 797 | 11 | 4.9 | 23 | 0 | 0 |
| 272 | 1130 | 21 | 9.7 | 21 | 0 | 0 |
| 212 | 884 | 12 | 5.6 | 26 | 0 | 0 |
| 254 | 1056 | 18 | 8.4 | 23 | 0 | 0 |
| 196 | 819 | 11 | 5 | 24 | 0 | 0 |
| 268 | 1114 | 20 | 9.4 | 22 | 0 | 0 |
| 624 | 2600 | 38 | 16.9 | 69 | 0 | 0 |
| 725 | 3013 | 52 | 23.9 | 63 | 0 | 0 |

MEAT &
MEAT DISHES

| MEAT DISHES | AVERAGE PORTION g |
|---|---|
| Beef bourguignon | 260 |
| Beef casserole, canned | 270 |
| Beef casserole, made with canned cook-in sauce | 300 |
| Beef hotpot with potatoes, shop bought | 260 |
| Beef stew | 280 |
| Beef stew, made with lean beef | 260 |
| Beef stew and dumplings | 260 |
| Cannelloni, shop bought | 260 |
| Chilli con carne | 220 |
| Chilli con carne, shop bought | 220 |
| Corned beef hash | 300 |
| Cottage pie | 310 |
| Cottage pie, shop bought | 310 |
| Irish stew | 330 |
| Irish stew, made with lean beef | 330 |
| Lamb hotpot with potatoes, shop bought | 260 |
| Lancashire hotpot | 260 |
| Lasagne, shop bought | 420 |
| Meatloaf | 100 |
| Moussaka | 330 |
| Moussaka, shop bought | 330 |
| Pork and beef meatballs in tomato sauce | 160 |
| Pork casserole, made with canned cook-in sauce | 260 |
| Sausage casserole | 350 |
| Shepherd's pie | 310 |
| Shepherd's pie, shop bought | 310 |
| Toad in the hole | 160 |
| Toad in the hole, made with skimmed milk and reduced-fat sausages | 160 |

Unless otherwise stated, all meat is lean and trimmed, and all chops and
cutlets are boned. Steaks are medium-sized. Unless stated otherwise, all
dishes are homemade.

| ENERGY kcal | ENERGY kJ | FAT g | SATURATED FAT g | PROTEIN g | CARBOHYDRATE g | FIBRE g |
|---|---|---|---|---|---|---|
| 328 | 1368 | 17 | 5.5 | 36 | 7 | 1 |
| 211 | 886 | 7 | 3.8 | 19 | 19 | 2.7 |
| | | | | | | |
| 408 | 1707 | 20 | 8.1 | 45 | 14 | 2.7 |
| 281 | 1183 | 11 | 4.4 | 19 | 28 | 2.3 |
| 316 | 1328 | 14 | 4.2 | 34 | 14 | 2 |
| 263 | 1102 | 9 | 2.3 | 32 | 13 | 1.8 |
| 499 | 2090 | 27 | 12.5 | 26 | 41 | 2.6 |
| 315 | 1326 | 13 | 5.2 | 17 | 35 | 3.1 |
| 286 | 1199 | 17 | 6.6 | 20 | 10 | 2.4 |
| 211 | 889 | 9 | 4.2 | 17 | 16 | 3.1 |
| 423 | 1776 | 18 | 9.9 | 31 | 37 | 3 |
| 391 | 1634 | 21 | 7.8 | 20 | 32 | 2.8 |
| 344 | 1448 | 17 | 7.4 | 14 | 37 | 2.8 |
| 399 | 1676 | 21 | 9.6 | 25 | 29 | 3.3 |
| 366 | 1541 | 17 | 7.3 | 26 | 29 | 3.3 |
| | | | | | | |
| 281 | 1183 | 11 | 4.4 | 19 | 28 | 2.3 |
| 289 | 1206 | 14 | 5.5 | 23 | 20 | 2.3 |
| 601 | 2533 | 26 | 11.8 | 31 | 66 | 2.9 |
| 214 | 894 | 11 | 4.1 | 17 | 13 | 0.5 |
| 403 | 1680 | 26 | 11.9 | 28 | 15 | 3.3 |
| 462 | 1934 | 27 | 9.6 | 27 | 28 | 2.6 |
| | | | | | | |
| 202 | 840 | 12 | 4.4 | 16 | 8 | 1.2 |
| | | | | | | |
| 398 | 1664 | 20 | 6.8 | 44 | 10 | 0 |
| 578 | 2405 | 38 | 12.3 | 42 | 18 | 3.1 |
| 391 | 1634 | 21 | 7.8 | 20 | 32 | 2.8 |
| 344 | 1448 | 17 | 7.4 | 14 | 37 | 2.8 |
| 443 | 1853 | 28 | 10.7 | 19 | 31 | 1.8 |
| | | | | | | |
| 320 | 1344 | 14 | 4.6 | 20 | 31 | 1.9 |

| MEAT PRODUCTS | AVERAGE PORTION g |
|---|---|
| Black pudding, dry-fried | 75 |
| Corned beef | 50 |
| Faggots in gravy, shop bought | 150 |
| Haggis, boiled | 85 |
| Luncheon meat, canned | 40 |
| Meatloaf, shop bought | 100 |
| Scotch eggs, shop bought | 120 |
| White pudding | 75 |

| SAUSAGES | |
|---|---|
| Beef sausages, fried | 40 |
| Beef sausages, grilled | 40 |
| Bratwurst | 75 |
| Chorizo | 30 |
| Frankfurter | 47 |
| Garlic sausage | 40 |
| Kabana | 30 |
| Mortadella | 24 |
| Pastrami | 50 |
| Pork and beef sausages, grilled | 40 |
| Pork and beef, economy sausages, fried | 40 |
| Pork and beef, economy sausages, grilled | 40 |
| Pork sausages, fried | 40 |
| Pork sausages, grilled | 40 |
| Pork sausages, frozen, fried | 40 |
| Pork sausages, frozen, grilled | 40 |
| Pork sausages, reduced-fat, fried | 40 |
| Pork sausages, reduced-fat, grilled | 40 |
| Premium sausages, fried | 40 |
| Premium sausages, grilled | 40 |
| Salami | 12 |
| Saveloy, unbattered, shop bought | 65 |

Unless otherwise stated, all meat is lean and trimmed, and all chops and cutlets are boned. Steaks are medium-sized. Unless stated otherwise, all dishes are homemade.

| ENERGY kcal | ENERGY kJ | FAT g | SATURATED FAT g | PROTEIN g | CARBOHYDRATE g | FIBRE g |
|---|---|---|---|---|---|---|
| 223 | 927 | 16 | 6.4 | 8 | 12 | 0.2 |
| 103 | 430 | 5 | 2.8 | 13 | 1 | 0 |
| 222 | 929 | 11 | 3.8 | 12 | 19 | 0.3 |
| 264 | 1098 | 18 | 6.5 | 9 | 16 | 0.2 |
| 112 | 463 | 10 | 3.5 | 5 | 1 | 0.1 |
| 216 | 900 | 16 | 5.6 | 17 | 1 | 0.5 |
| 301 | 1255 | 5.2 | 19 | 14 | 16 | 0 |
| 338 | 1407 | 24 | 8 | 5 | 27 | 1 |
| | | | | | | |
| 112 | 464 | 8 | 3 | 5 | 5 | 0.3 |
| 111 | 463 | 8 | 3.2 | 5 | 5 | 0.3 |
| 195 | 811 | 16 | 6 | 12 | 2 | Trace |
| 87 | 362 | 7 | 2.9 | 5 | 1 | Trace |
| 135 | 559 | 12 | 4.3 | 6 | 1 | 0 |
| 99 | 412 | 8 | 2.9 | 6 | 0 | Trace |
| 92 | 383 | 8 | 3.4 | 5 | 0 | Trace |
| 79 | 328 | 7 | 2.8 | 3 | 0 | Trace |
| 62 | 259 | 2 | 0.9 | 10 | 1 | 0 |
| 108 | 448 | 8 | 3 | 5 | 4 | 0.5 |
| 99 | 414 | 7 | 1.8 | 5 | 5 | 0.5 |
| | | | | | | |
| 103 | 429 | 7 | 1.9 | 5 | 5 | 0.5 |
| 123 | 512 | 10 | 3.4 | 6 | 4 | 0.3 |
| 118 | 488 | 9 | 3.2 | 6 | 4 | 0.3 |
| 126 | 525 | 10 | 3.5 | 6 | 4 | 0.3 |
| 116 | 482 | 8 | 3 | 6 | 4 | 0.3 |
| 84 | 352 | 5 | 1.7 | 6 | 4 | 0.6 |
| 92 | 384 | 6 | 2 | 6 | 4 | 0.6 |
| 110 | 457 | 8 | 3.1 | 6 | 3 | 0.3 |
| 117 | 486 | 9 | 3.3 | 7 | 3 | 0.3 |
| 53 | 218 | 5 | 1.8 | 3 | 0 | 0 |
| 192 | 801 | 18 | 3.6 | 9 | 7 | 0.5 |

MEAT &
MEAT DISHES 43

| | AVERAGE PORTION g |
|---|---|
| **BEEFBURGERS** | |
| Beefburgers, fried | 36 |
| Beefburgers, grilled | 100 |
| Beefburgers, fried | 100 |
| Beefburgers, grilled | 100 |
| Beefburgers, low-fat, fried | 100 |
| Beefburgers, low-fat, grilled | 100 |
| Beefburgers in gravy, canned | 100 |
| | |
| **PIES AND PASTIES** | |
| Beef pie, shop bought | 141 |
| Cornish pasty | 155 |
| Cornish pasty, shop bought | 155 |
| Lamb samosa, baked | 70 |
| Lamb samosa, deep-fried | 70 |
| Pork and egg pie | 60 |
| Pork pie | 60 |
| Pork pie, mini | 50 |
| Sausage rolls, flaky pastry | 60 |
| Sausage rolls, shortcrust pastry | 60 |
| Steak and kidney pie, double crust | 120 |
| Steak and kidney pie, shop bought | 141 |
| | |
| **OFFAL** | |
| Heart, lamb, roasted | 200 |
| Heart, lamb, stewed | 200 |
| Heart, ox, stewed | 200 |
| Heart, pig, stewed | 100 |
| Kidney, lamb, fried | 35 |
| Kidney, ox, stewed | 112 |
| Kidney, pig, fried | 140 |
| Kidney, pig, stewed | 140 |
| Liver, calf, fried | 100 |

Unless otherwise stated, all meat is lean and trimmed, and all chops and
cutlets are boned. Steaks are medium-sized. Unless stated otherwise, all
dishes are homemade.

| ENERGY kcal | ENERGY kJ | FAT g | SATURATED FAT g | PROTEIN g | CARBOHYDRATE g | FIBRE g |
|---|---|---|---|---|---|---|
| 118 | 493 | 9 | 3.9 | 10 | 0 | 0 |
| 326 | 1355 | 24 | 10.9 | 27 | 0 | 0 |
| 303 | 1261 | 23 | 8.7 | 24 | 1 | 0.2 |
| 287 | 1194 | 20 | 8.8 | 25 | 1 | 0.2 |
| 193 | 807 | 11 | 5 | 24 | 0 | 0 |
| 178 | 745 | 10 | 4.4 | 23 | 1 | 0 |
| 171 | 713 | 12 | 4.8 | 12 | 5 | Trace |
| 437 | 1826 | 24 | 11.8 | 12 | 38 | 0.7 |
| 456 | 1905 | 28 | 9.8 | 10 | 43 | 2.6 |
| 414 | 1731 | 25 | 9.1 | 10 | 39 | 1.4 |
| 187 | 781 | 10 | 2.5 | 8 | 16 | 1.2 |
| 265 | 1097 | 22 | 3.3 | 6 | 12 | 0.8 |
| 178 | 740 | 13 | 4.4 | 6 | 10 | 0.5 |
| 228 | 947 | 18 | 6.8 | 6 | 11 | 0.5 |
| 196 | 815 | 14 | 5.7 | 5 | 13 | 0.5 |
| 238 | 991 | 17 | 6.5 | 6 | 15 | 0.8 |
| 229 | 953 | 16 | 5.8 | 6 | 17 | 0.9 |
| 406 | 1694 | 26 | 9.7 | 16 | 27 | 1.1 |
| 437 | 1826 | 24 | 11.8 | 12 | 38 | 0.7 |
| 452 | 1888 | 28 | 6.2 | 51 | 0 | 0 |
| 312 | 1308 | 15 | 6 | 24 | 20 | 0 |
| 314 | 1322 | 10 | 5 | 56 | 0 | 0 |
| 162 | 678 | 7 | 1.3 | 25 | 0 | 0 |
| 66 | 274 | 4 | 0.4 | 8 | 0 | 0 |
| 155 | 648 | 5 | 1.6 | 27 | 0 | 0 |
| 283 | 1187 | 13 | 2.1 | 41 | 0 | 0 |
| 214 | 897 | 9 | 2.8 | 34 | 0 | 0 |
| 176 | 734 | 10 | 2.7 | 22 | Trace | 0 |

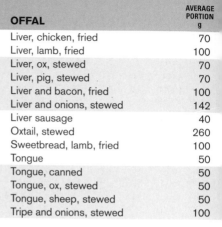

| OFFAL | AVERAGE PORTION g |
|---|---|
| Liver, chicken, fried | 70 |
| Liver, lamb, fried | 100 |
| Liver, ox, stewed | 70 |
| Liver, pig, stewed | 70 |
| Liver and bacon, fried | 100 |
| Liver and onions, stewed | 142 |
| Liver sausage | 40 |
| Oxtail, stewed | 260 |
| Sweetbread, lamb, fried | 100 |
| Tongue | 50 |
| Tongue, canned | 50 |
| Tongue, ox, stewed | 50 |
| Tongue, sheep, stewed | 50 |
| Tripe and onions, stewed | 100 |

## PORK, BACON AND HAM

### Bacon

| | |
|---|---|
| Collar joint, boiled | 46 |
| Collar joint, untrimmed, boiled | 46 |
| Loin steaks, grilled | 100 |
| Rashers, back, dry-cured, grilled | 100 |
| Rashers, back, dry-fried | 100 |
| Rashers, back, grilled | 100 |
| Rashers, back, untrimmed, grilled | 100 |
| Rashers, back, grilled crispy | 100 |
| Rashers, back, reduced salt, grilled | 100 |
| Rashers, back, smoked, grilled | 100 |
| Rashers, back, sweetcure, grilled | 100 |
| Rashers, back, 'tendersweet', grilled | 100 |
| Rashers, middle, fried | 100 |
| Rashers, middle, grilled | 100 |
| Rashers, streaky, fried | 100 |
| Rashers, streaky, grilled | 100 |

Unless otherwise stated, all meat is lean and trimmed, and all chops and cutlets are boned. Steaks are medium-sized. Unless stated otherwise, all dishes are homemade.

| ENERGY kcal | ENERGY kJ | FAT g | SATURATED FAT g | PROTEIN g | CARBOHYDRATE g | FIBRE g |
|---|---|---|---|---|---|---|
| 118 | 494 | 6 | 3.5 | 15 | Trace | 0 |
| 237 | 989 | 13 | 4.9 | 30 | Trace | 0 |
| 139 | 582 | 7 | 2.5 | 17 | 2 | 0 |
| 132 | 555 | 6 | 1.8 | 18 | 2 | 0 |
| 247 | 1030 | 15 | 2.1 | 29 | Trace | 0 |
| 210 | 879 | 11 | 2.1 | 21 | 8 | 1.4 |
| 90 | 377 | 7 | 2.1 | 5 | 2 | 0.3 |
| 632 | 2636 | 35 | 12 | 79 | 0 | 0 |
| 217 | 910 | 11 | 5 | 29 | 0 | 0 |
| 101 | 418 | 7 | 3 | 9 | Trace | Trace |
| 107 | 442 | 8 | 3.2 | 8 | Trace | 0 |
| 121 | 504 | 9 | 3 | 10 | 0 | 0 |
| 145 | 599 | 12 | 5 | 9 | 0 | 0 |
| 93 | 393 | 3 | 1.5 | 8 | 10 | 0.7 |
| | | | | | | |
| 88 | 368 | 4 | 1.7 | 12 | 0 | 0 |
| 150 | 619 | 12 | 4.9 | 9 | 0 | 0 |
| 191 | 799 | 10 | 3.5 | 26 | 0 | 0 |
| 257 | 1071 | 16 | 6 | 28 | 0 | 0 |
| 295 | 1225 | 22 | 8.3 | 24 | 0 | 0 |
| 214 | 892 | 12 | 4.6 | 26 | 0 | 0 |
| 287 | 1194 | 22 | 8.1 | 23 | 0 | 0 |
| 313 | 1308 | 19 | 7.1 | 36 | 0 | 0 |
| 282 | 1172 | 21 | 7.8 | 24 | 0 | 0 |
| 293 | 1216 | 22 | 8.3 | 23 | 0 | 0 |
| 258 | 1074 | 17 | 6.6 | 24 | 2 | 0 |
| 213 | 889 | 12 | 4.5 | 26 | Trace | 0 |
| 350 | 1452 | 29 | 9.8 | 23 | 0 | 0 |
| 307 | 1276 | 23 | 8.4 | 25 | 0 | 0 |
| 335 | 1389 | 27 | 9.1 | 24 | 0 | 0 |
| 337 | 1400 | 27 | 9.8 | 24 | 0 | 0 |

MEAT &

## PORK, BACON AND HAM

| | AVERAGE PORTION g |
|---|---|
| Belly joint, untrimmed, roasted | 110 |
| Belly, untrimmed, grilled | 110 |
| Chump chops, untrimmed, fried | 170 |
| Chump steaks, untrimmed, fried | 170 |
| Crackling, cooked | 50 |
| Fillet, grilled, lean | 120 |
| Fillet, untrimmed, grilled | 120 |
| Fillet strips, stir-fried, lean | 90 |
| **Gammon** | |
| Joint, boiled | 170 |
| Rashers, grilled | 100 |
| **Ham** | |
| Ham, canned | 90 |
| Ham, Parma | 47 |
| Ham, premium | 56 |
| Pork shoulder, cured | 100 |
| Kebabs, grilled | 90 |
| Kebabs, untrimmed, grilled | 90 |
| Leg joint, untrimmed, frozen, roasted | 90 |
| Leg joint, roasted medium | 90 |
| Leg joint, untrimmed, roasted medium | 90 |
| Leg joint, roasted well done | 90 |
| Leg joint, untrimmed, roasted well done | 90 |
| Loin chops, grilled | 75 |
| Loin chops, untrimmed, grilled | 75 |
| Loin chops, grilled | 120 |
| Loin chops, untrimmed, grilled | 120 |
| Loin chops, roasted | 75 |
| Loin chops, untrimmed, roasted | 75 |
| Loin joint, pot roasted | 90 |
| Loin joint, untrimmed, pot roasted | 90 |
| Loin joint, roasted | 90 |
| Loin joint, untrimmed, roasted | 90 |
| Loin steaks, fried | 120 |

Unless otherwise stated, all meat is lean and trimmed, and all chops and cutlets are boned. Steaks are medium-sized. Unless stated otherwise, all dishes are homemade.

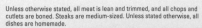

| ENERGY kcal | ENERGY kJ | FAT g | SATURATED FAT g | PROTEIN g | CARBOHYDRATE g | FIBRE g |
|---|---|---|---|---|---|---|
| 322 | 1341 | 24 | 8.1 | 28 | 0 | 0 |
| 352 | 1465 | 26 | 9 | 30 | 0 | 0 |
| 498 | 2069 | 37 | 11.9 | 42 | 0 | 0 |
| 369 | 1542 | 20 | 6.3 | 47 | 0 | 0 |
| 275 | 1140 | 23 | 7.7 | 18 | 0 | 0 |
| 204 | 863 | 5 | 1.8 | 40 | 0 | 0 |
| 214 | 899 | 6 | 2.3 | 40 | 0 | 0 |
| 164 | 688 | 5 | 1.2 | 29 | 0 | 0 |
| | | | | | | |
| 347 | 1447 | 21 | 7 | 40 | 0 | 0 |
| 199 | 834 | 10 | 3.4 | 28 | 0 | 0 |
| | | | | | | |
| 96 | 404 | 4 | 1.4 | 15 | 0 | 0 |
| 105 | 438 | 6 | 2 | 13 | Trace | Trace |
| 74 | 310 | 3 | 1 | 12 | 0 | 0 |
| 103 | 435 | 4 | 1.2 | 17 | 1 | 0 |
| 161 | 679 | 4 | 1.4 | 31 | 0 | 0 |
| 170 | 717 | 5 | 2 | 30 | 0 | 0 |
| 202 | 842 | 10 | 3.6 | 28 | 0 | 0 |
| 164 | 689 | 5 | 1.7 | 30 | 0 | 0 |
| 194 | 813 | 9 | 3.2 | 28 | 0 | 0 |
| 167 | 701 | 5 | 1.6 | 31 | 0 | 0 |
| 233 | 974 | 14 | 4.9 | 27 | 0 | 0 |
| 140 | 585 | 5 | 1.8 | 23 | 0 | 0 |
| 191 | 800 | 12 | 4.3 | 21 | 0 | 0 |
| 221 | 929 | 8 | 2.6 | 38 | 0 | 0 |
| 308 | 1289 | 19 | 6.7 | 35 | 0 | 0 |
| 181 | 758 | 8 | 2.8 | 28 | 0 | 0 |
| 226 | 942 | 14 | 5.3 | 24 | 0 | 0 |
| 177 | 744 | 7 | 2.6 | 28 | 0 | 0 |
| 275 | 1142 | 21 | 7.4 | 22 | 0 | 0 |
| 164 | 687 | 6 | 2.2 | 27 | 0 | 0 |
| 228 | 949 | 15 | 5.3 | 24 | 0 | 0 |
| 229 | 962 | 9 | 2.8 | 38 | 0 | 0 |

MEAT &
MEAT DISHES

## PORK, BACON AND HAM

| | AVERAGE PORTION g |
|---|---|
| Loin steaks, untrimmed, fried | 120 |
| Mince, stewed | 90 |
| Pork, diced, casseroled | 90 |
| Pork, diced, untrimmed, casseroled | 90 |
| Pork steaks, grilled | 135 |
| Pork steaks, untrimmed, grilled | 135 |
| Pork steaks, stewed | 135 |
| Pork steaks, untrimmed, stewed | 135 |
| Spare rib, untrimmed, grilled | 110 |
| Spare rib chops, braised | 140 |
| Spare rib chops, untrimmed, braised | 140 |
| Spare rib joint, pot roasted | 90 |
| Spare rib joint, untrimmed, pot roasted | 90 |

Unless otherwise stated, all meat is lean and trimmed, and all chops and
cutlets are boned. Steaks are medium-sized. Unless stated otherwise, all
dishes are homemade.

| ENERGY kcal | ENERGY kJ | FAT g | SATURATED FAT g | PROTEIN g | CARBOHYDRATE g | FIBRE g |
|---|---|---|---|---|---|---|
| 331 | 1378 | 22 | 7.2 | 33 | 0 | 0 |
| 172 | 720 | 9 | 3.5 | 22 | 0 | 0 |
| 166 | 698 | 6 | 1.7 | 29 | 0 | 0 |
| 166 | 698 | 6 | 1.8 | 28 | 0 | 0 |
| 228 | 963 | 5 | 1.8 | 46 | 0 | 0 |
| 267 | 1123 | 10 | 3.6 | 44 | 0 | 0 |
| 238 | 1000 | 6 | 1.8 | 45 | 0 | 0 |
| 269 | 1126 | 11 | 3.2 | 42 | 0 | 0 |
| 321 | 1340 | 21 | 8.3 | 32 | 0 | 0 |
| 298 | 1249 | 14 | 5 | 43 | 0 | 0 |
| 346 | 1446 | 21 | 7.7 | 39 | 0 | 0 |
| 181 | 759 | 8 | 2.9 | 27 | 0 | 0 |
| 234 | 973 | 16 | 6 | 22 | 0 | 0 |

MEAT &
MEAT DISHES 51

| CHICKEN | AVERAGE PORTION g |
|---|---|
| Breast, casseroled | 130 |
| Breast, skinned, casseroled | 130 |
| Breast, grilled | 130 |
| Breast, grilled and skinned | 130 |
| Breast, skinned, grilled | 130 |
| Breast strips, stir-fried | 90 |
| Corn-fed chicken, roasted, dark meat | 90 |
| Corn-fed chicken, roasted, light meat | 90 |
| Dark meat, roasted | 100 |
| Drumsticks, casseroled | 47 |
| Drumsticks, skinned, casseroled | 47 |
| Drumsticks, roasted | 47 |
| Drumsticks, skinned, roasted | 47 |
| Leg quarter, casseroled | 146 |
| Leg quarter, skinned, casseroled | 146 |
| Leg quarter, roasted | 146 |
| Light meat, roasted | 100 |
| Thighs, casseroled | 45 |
| Thighs, skinned, boned and diced, casseroled | 45 |
| Wing quarter, casseroled | 150 |
| Wing quarter, skinned, casseroled | 150 |
| Wing quarter, roasted | 150 |
| Wings, grilled | 100 |

### CHICKEN PRODUCTS

| | |
|---|---|
| Chicken fingers, baked | 90 |
| Chicken goujons, baked | 90 |
| Chicken in crumbs, stuffed with cheese and vegetables, baked | 100 |
| Chicken in white sauce, canned | 100 |
| Chicken Kiev, frozen, baked | 170 |

Unless otherwise stated, chicken and turkey are neither skinned nor boned, game is skinned and trimmed and dishes are homemade.

| ENERGY kcal | ENERGY kJ | FAT g | SATURATED FAT g | PROTEIN g | CARBOHYDRATE g | FIBRE g |
|---|---|---|---|---|---|---|
| 239 | 1004 | 11 | 3.1 | 35 | 0 | 0 |
| 148 | 628 | 7 | 2 | 37 | 0 | 0 |
| 225 | 946 | 8 | 1.2 | 38 | 0 | 0 |
| 191 | 807 | 4 | 1.2 | 39 | 0 | 0 |
| 192 | 814 | 4 | 0.8 | 42 | 0 | 0 |
| 145 | 609 | 4 | 0.8 | 27 | 0 | 0 |
| 167 | 695 | 9 | 2.5 | 22 | 0 | 0 |
| 127 | 536 | 4 | 1.1 | 23 | 0 | 0 |
| 196 | 819 | 11 | 2.9 | 24 | 0 | 0 |
| 102 | 425 | 7 | 1.8 | 10 | 0 | 0 |
| 87 | 363 | 5 | 1.2 | 11 | 0 | 0 |
| 87 | 364 | 4 | 1.2 | 12 | 0 | 0 |
| 71 | 301 | 2 | 0.7 | 13 | 0 | 0 |
| 317 | 1320 | 20 | 5.5 | 33 | 0 | 0 |
| 257 | 1075 | 12 | 3.4 | 37 | 0 | 0 |
| 345 | 1432 | 25 | 6.7 | 31 | 0 | 0 |
| 153 | 645 | 4 | 1 | 30 | 0 | 0 |
| 105 | 436 | 7 | 2 | 10 | 0 | 0 |
| 81 | 340 | 4 | 1.1 | 12 | 0 | 0 |
| 315 | 1316 | 19 | 5.3 | 37 | 0 | 0 |
| 246 | 1035 | 9 | 2.6 | 40 | 0 | 0 |
| 339 | 1415 | 21 | 5.9 | 37 | 0 | 0 |
| 274 | 1146 | 17 | 4.6 | 27 | Trace | 0 |
| 185 | 774 | 9 | 2.7 | 11 | 17 | Trace |
| 249 | 1045 | 13 | 3.6 | 17 | 18 | 0.6 |
| 230 | 963 | 14 | 4.1 | 16 | 11 | 0.9 |
| 141 | 590 | 8 | 2.3 | 14 | 3 | Trace |
| 456 | 1902 | 29 | 12.1 | 32 | 19 | 1 |

POULTRY
& GAME 53

### CHICKEN PRODUCTS

| | AVERAGE PORTION g |
|---|---|
| Chicken pancakes, frozen, shallow-fried | 100 |
| Chicken roll | 24 |
| Chicken slices | 80 |

### CHICKEN PIES

| | |
|---|---|
| Chicken and mushroom pie, single crust | 100 |
| Chicken pie, individual, baked | 130 |

### CHICKEN DISHES

| | |
|---|---|
| Chicken chasseur | 260 |
| Chicken in sauce with vegetables | 290 |
| Chicken curry | 350 |
| Chicken curry, with bone | 350 |
| Chicken curry, without bone | 300 |
| Chicken fricassée | 200 |
| Chicken in white sauce, made with semi-skimmed milk | 200 |
| Chicken in white sauce, made with whole milk | 200 |
| Chicken risotto | 350 |
| Coronation chicken | 200 |
| Lemon chicken | 100 |
| Tandoori chicken | 100 |

Unless otherwise stated, chicken and turkey are neither skinned nor boned, game is skinned and trimmed and dishes are homemade.

| ENERGY kcal | ENERGY kJ | FAT g | SATURATED FAT g | PROTEIN g | CARBOHYDRATE g | FIBRE g |
|---|---|---|---|---|---|---|
| 260 | 1090 | 14 | 1.4 | 6 | 29 | 0.1 |
| 31 | 132 | 1 | 0.4 | 4 | 1 | Trace |
| 91 | 386 | 1 | 0.3 | 19 | 2 | 0 |
| | | | | | | |
| 200 | 836 | 10 | 4.5 | 13 | 14 | 0.6 |
| 374 | 1563 | 21 | 9.1 | 12 | 32 | 1 |
| | | | | | | |
| 203 | 861 | 5 | 0.8 | 33 | 7 | 0.8 |
| 336 | 1412 | 15 | 7 | 39 | 13 | 0.9 |
| 522 | 2174 | 31 | 14 | 42 | 19 | 4.5 |
| 539 | 2237 | 44 | 6 | 27 | 8 | 2.4 |
| 615 | 2550 | 51 | 6.6 | 31 | 9 | 2.7 |
| 214 | 896 | 12 | 4.8 | 22 | 6 | 1 |
| 310 | 1298 | 16 | 5 | 34 | 10 | 0.2 |
| 328 | 1376 | 18 | 6.2 | 34 | 10 | 0.2 |
| 546 | 2310 | 10 | 4.5 | 31 | 84 | Trace |
| 728 | 3012 | 63 | 10.4 | 33 | 6 | Trace |
| 155 | 652 | 6 | 0.8 | 16 | 9 | Trace |
| 214 | 897 | 11 | 3.3 | 27 | 2 | Trace |

## GAME

| | AVERAGE PORTION g |
|---|---|
| Duck, roasted | 185 |
| Duck, untrimmed, roasted | 185 |
| Goose, roasted | 185 |
| Goose, untrimmed, roasted | 185 |
| Grouse, roasted | 160 |
| Pheasant, roasted | 160 |
| Pigeon, roasted | 115 |
| Rabbit, stewed | 160 |
| Venison, roasted | 120 |

## TURKEY

| | |
|---|---|
| Breast, grilled and skinned | 90 |
| Dark meat, roasted | 90 |
| Drumsticks, roasted | 90 |
| Drumsticks, roasted and skinned | 90 |
| Light meat, from self-basting bird, roasted | 90 |
| Light meat, roasted | 90 |
| Mince, stewed | 90 |
| Strips, stir-fried | 90 |
| Thighs, diced, skinned, boned, casseroled | 90 |

Unless otherwise stated, chicken and turkey are neither skinned nor
boned, game is skinned and trimmed and dishes are homemade.

| ENERGY kcal | ENERGY kJ | FAT g | SATURATED FAT g | PROTEIN g | CARBOHYDRATE g | FIBRE g |
|---|---|---|---|---|---|---|
| 361 | 1508 | 19 | 6.1 | 47 | 0 | 0 |
| 783 | 3238 | 92 | 21.1 | 37 | 0 | 0 |
| 590 | 2455 | 41 | 13.7 | 54 | 0 | 0 |
| 557 | 2316 | 39 | 12.2 | 51 | 0 | 0 |
| 205 | 869 | 3 | 0.8 | 44 | 0 | 0 |
| 352 | 1469 | 5 | 0.6 | 45 | 0 | 0 |
| 215 | 903 | 9 | 3 | 33 | 0 | 0 |
| 182 | 766 | 5 | 2.7 | 34 | 0 | 0 |
| 198 | 838 | 3 | 1 | 43 | 0 | 0 |
| | | | | | | |
| 140 | 592 | 2 | 0.5 | 32 | 0 | 0 |
| 159 | 671 | 6 | 1.8 | 26 | 0 | 0 |
| 167 | 702 | 8 | 2.3 | 25 | 0 | 0 |
| 146 | 615 | 5 | 1.5 | 25 | 0 | 0 |
| 147 | 619 | 4 | 1.1 | 29 | 0 | 0 |
| 138 | 583 | 2 | 0.6 | 30 | 0 | 0 |
| 158 | 665 | 6 | 1.8 | 26 | 0 | 0 |
| 148 | 623 | 4 | 1.1 | 28 | 0 | 0 |
| 163 | 684 | 7 | 2.3 | 25 | 0 | 0 |

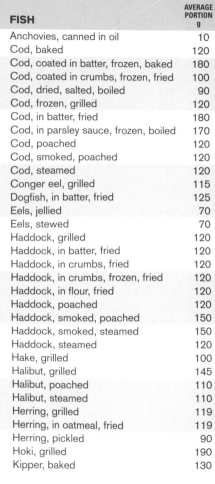

| FISH | AVERAGE PORTION g |
|---|---|
| Anchovies, canned in oil | 10 |
| Cod, baked | 120 |
| Cod, coated in batter, frozen, baked | 180 |
| Cod, coated in crumbs, frozen, fried | 100 |
| Cod, dried, salted, boiled | 90 |
| Cod, frozen, grilled | 120 |
| Cod, in batter, fried | 180 |
| Cod, in parsley sauce, frozen, boiled | 170 |
| Cod, poached | 120 |
| Cod, smoked, poached | 120 |
| Cod, steamed | 120 |
| Conger eel, grilled | 115 |
| Dogfish, in batter, fried | 125 |
| Eels, jellied | 70 |
| Eels, stewed | 70 |
| Haddock, grilled | 120 |
| Haddock, in batter, fried | 120 |
| Haddock, in crumbs, fried | 120 |
| Haddock, in crumbs, frozen, fried | 120 |
| Haddock, in flour, fried | 120 |
| Haddock, poached | 120 |
| Haddock, smoked, poached | 150 |
| Haddock, smoked, steamed | 150 |
| Haddock, steamed | 120 |
| Hake, grilled | 100 |
| Halibut, grilled | 145 |
| Halibut, poached | 110 |
| Halibut, steamed | 110 |
| Herring, grilled | 119 |
| Herring, in oatmeal, fried | 119 |
| Herring, pickled | 90 |
| Hoki, grilled | 190 |
| Kipper, baked | 130 |

Unless otherwise stated, values for bottled and canned seafood are for drained weights.

| ENERGY kcal | ENERGY kJ | FAT g | SATURATED FAT g | PROTEIN g | CARBOHYDRATE g | FIBRE g |
|---|---|---|---|---|---|---|
| 28 | 117 | 2 | 0.4 | 3 | 0 | 0 |
| 115 | 490 | 1 | 0.4 | 26 | Trace | 0 |
| 380 | 1589 | 21 | 6.5 | 23 | 26 | 1.1 |
| 235 | 983 | 14 | 1.5 | 12 | 15 | 0.4 |
| 124 | 527 | 1 | 0.2 | 29 | 0 | 0 |
| 114 | 482 | 2 | 0.5 | 25 | Trace | 0 |
| 445 | 1856 | 28 | 7.4 | 29 | 21 | 0.9 |
| 143 | 598 | 5 | 3 | 20 | 5 | 0.2 |
| 113 | 475 | 1 | 0.4 | 25 | Trace | 0 |
| 121 | 511 | 2 | 0.7 | 26 | Trace | 0 |
| 100 | 420 | 1 | 0.2 | 22 | 0 | 0 |
| 158 | 660 | 6 | Trace | 25 | 0 | 0 |
| 369 | 1531 | 27 | 6.6 | 18 | 13 | 0.5 |
| 69 | 284 | 5 | 1.3 | 6 | Trace | 0 |
| 141 | 589 | 9 | 1.3 | 14 | 0 | 0 |
| 125 | 530 | 1 | 0.2 | 29 | 0 | 0 |
| 278 | 1163 | 17 | 4.4 | 21 | 12 | 0.5 |
| 209 | 875 | 10 | 0.8 | 26 | 4 | 0.2 |
| 235 | 986 | 12 | 1 | 18 | 15 | 0.7 |
| 166 | 698 | 5 | 0.5 | 25 | 5 | 0.2 |
| 136 | 572 | 5 | 3.1 | 21 | 1 | 0 |
| 201 | 843 | 9 | 5.6 | 28 | 2 | 0 |
| 152 | 644 | 1 | 0.3 | 35 | 0 | 0 |
| 107 | 454 | 1 | 0.1 | 25 | 0 | 0 |
| 113 | 478 | 3 | 0.4 | 22 | 0 | 0 |
| 175 | 744 | 3 | 0.6 | 37 | 0 | 0 |
| 169 | 713 | 6 | 3 | 27 | 1 | 0 |
| 144 | 608 | 4 | 0.6 | 26 | 0 | 0 |
| 215 | 900 | 13 | 3.3 | 24 | 0 | 0 |
| 278 | 1160 | 18 | 3.3 | 27 | 2 | 0.1 |
| 188 | 789 | 10 | 3.3 | 15 | 9 | 0 |
| 230 | 969 | 5 | 1 | 46 | 0 | 0 |
| 267 | 1112 | 15 | 2.3 | 33 | 0 | 0 |

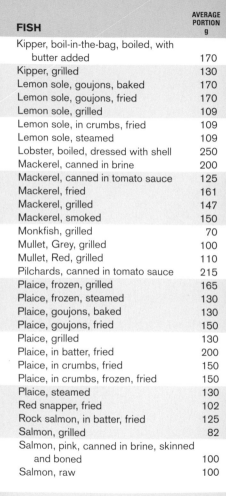

| FISH | AVERAGE PORTION g |
|---|---|
| Kipper, boil-in-the-bag, boiled, with butter added | 170 |
| Kipper, grilled | 130 |
| Lemon sole, goujons, baked | 170 |
| Lemon sole, goujons, fried | 170 |
| Lemon sole, grilled | 109 |
| Lemon sole, in crumbs, fried | 109 |
| Lemon sole, steamed | 109 |
| Lobster, boiled, dressed with shell | 250 |
| Mackerel, canned in brine | 200 |
| Mackerel, canned in tomato sauce | 125 |
| Mackerel, fried | 161 |
| Mackerel, grilled | 147 |
| Mackerel, smoked | 150 |
| Monkfish, grilled | 70 |
| Mullet, Grey, grilled | 100 |
| Mullet, Red, grilled | 110 |
| Pilchards, canned in tomato sauce | 215 |
| Plaice, frozen, grilled | 165 |
| Plaice, frozen, steamed | 130 |
| Plaice, goujons, baked | 130 |
| Plaice, goujons, fried | 150 |
| Plaice, grilled | 130 |
| Plaice, in batter, fried | 200 |
| Plaice, in crumbs, fried | 150 |
| Plaice, in crumbs, frozen, fried | 150 |
| Plaice, steamed | 130 |
| Red snapper, fried | 102 |
| Rock salmon, in batter, fried | 125 |
| Salmon, grilled | 82 |
| Salmon, pink, canned in brine, skinned and boned | 100 |
| Salmon, raw | 100 |

Unless otherwise stated, values for bottled and canned seafood are for drained weights.

| ENERGY kcal | ENERGY kJ | FAT g | SATURATED FAT g | PROTEIN g | CARBOHYDRATE g | FIBRE g |
|---|---|---|---|---|---|---|
| 403 | 1673 | 30 | 2.7 | 34 | Trace | 0 |
| 332 | 1378 | 25 | 4 | 26 | 0 | 0 |
| 318 | 1318 | 25 | Trace | 27 | 25 | Trace |
| 636 | 2640 | 49 | 5.4 | 26 | 24 | Trace |
| 106 | 445 | 2 | 0.2 | 22 | 0 | 0 |
| 235 | 985 | 14 | 1.4 | 18 | 10 | 0.4 |
| 99 | 419 | 1 | 0.1 | 22 | 0 | 0 |
| 258 | 1088 | 4 | 0.5 | 55 | Trace | 0 |
| 474 | 1970 | 36 | 8 | 38 | 0 | 0 |
| 258 | 1070 | 19 | 4.1 | 20 | 2 | Trace |
| 438 | 1819 | 31 | 6.4 | 39 | 0 | 0 |
| 351 | 1461 | 25 | 5.1 | 31 | 0 | 0 |
| 531 | 2198 | 46 | 9.5 | 28 | 0 | 0 |
| 67 | 285 | 0 | 0.1 | 16 | 0 | 0 |
| 150 | 629 | 5 | 1.4 | 26 | 0 | 0 |
| 133 | 561 | 5 | 1.4 | 22 | 0 | 0 |
| 310 | 1292 | 17 | 3.7 | 36 | 2 | Trace |
| 200 | 843 | 3 | 0.5 | 42 | 0 | 0 |
| 120 | 506 | 2 | 0.3 | 25 | 0 | 0 |
| 395 | 1651 | 24 | 0 | 11 | 36 | Trace |
| 639 | 2657 | 48 | 5.4 | 13 | 41 | Trace |
| 125 | 525 | 2 | 0.4 | 26 | 0 | 0 |
| 514 | 2144 | 34 | 9 | 30 | 24 | 1 |
| 342 | 1427 | 21 | 2.3 | 27 | 13 | 0.3 |
| 261 | 1094 | 14 | 1.5 | 21 | 14 | 0.5 |
| 121 | 510 | 2 | 0.4 | 25 | 0 | 0 |
| 129 | 542 | 3 | 0.7 | 25 | 0 | 0 |
| 369 | 1531 | 27 | 6.6 | 18 | 13 | 0.5 |
| 176 | 735 | 11 | 2.1 | 20 | 0 | 0 |
| 153 | 644 | 7 | 1.3 | 24 | 0 | 0 |
| 180 | 750 | 11 | 1.9 | 20 | 0 | 0 |

| **FISH** | AVERAGE PORTION g |
|---|---|
| Salmon, red, canned in brine, skinned and boned | 100 |
| Salmon, smoked | 56 |
| Salmon, steamed | 77 |
| Sardines, canned in brine | 100 |
| Sardines, canned in oil | 100 |
| Sardines, canned in tomato sauce | 100 |
| Sardines, grilled | 40 |
| Skate, grilled | 215 |
| Skate, in batter, fried | 170 |
| Sprats, fried | 132 |
| Swordfish, grilled | 125 |
| Trout, brown, steamed | 155 |
| Trout, rainbow, grilled | 155 |
| Tuna, canned in brine | 45 |
| Tuna, canned in oil | 45 |
| Tuna, raw | 45 |
| Whitebait, in flour, fried | 80 |
| Whiting, in crumbs, fried | 162 |
| Whiting, steamed | 85 |

| **FISH PRODUCTS AND DISHES** | |
|---|---|
| Caviare, bottled in brine | 19 |
| Fish balls, steamed | 50 |
| Fish cakes, fried | 100 |
| Fish cakes, grilled | 100 |
| Fish cakes, salmon, grilled | 100 |
| Fish fingers, cod, fried | 56 |
| Fish fingers, cod, grilled | 56 |
| Fish paste | 10 |
| Fisherman's pie, shop bought | 170 |
| Kedgeree | 300 |
| Mackerel pâté, smoked | 40 |

Unless otherwise stated, values for bottled and canned seafood are for drained weights. Dishes are homemade unless otherwise stated.

| ENERGY kcal | ENERGY kJ | FAT g | SATURATED FAT g | PROTEIN g | CARBOHYDRATE g | FIBRE g |
|---|---|---|---|---|---|---|
| 167 | 700 | 8 | 1.7 | 22 | 0 | 0 |
| 80 | 335 | 3 | 0.4 | 14 | 0 | 0 |
| 152 | 634 | 10 | 1.8 | 15 | 0 | 0 |
| 172 | 721 | 10 | 2.8 | 22 | 0 | 0 |
| 220 | 918 | 14 | 2.9 | 23 | 0 | 0 |
| 162 | 678 | 10 | 2.8 | 17 | 1 | Trace |
| 78 | 326 | 4 | 1.2 | 10 | 0 | 0 |
| 170 | 725 | 1 | 0.2 | 41 | 0 | 0 |
| 286 | 1193 | 17 | 4.3 | 25 | 8 | 0.3 |
| 548 | 2268 | 46 | 7 | 33 | 0 | 0 |
| 174 | 729 | 6 | 1.5 | 29 | 0 | 0 |
| 209 | 877 | 7 | 1.6 | 36 | 0 | 0 |
| 209 | 876 | 8 | 1.7 | 33 | 0 | 0 |
| 45 | 190 | 1 | 0.1 | 11 | 0 | 0 |
| 85 | 357 | 4 | 0.7 | 12 | 0 | 0 |
| 61 | 258 | 2 | 0.5 | 11 | 0 | 0 |
| 420 | 1739 | 38 | 2.1 | 16 | 4 | 0.2 |
| 309 | 1298 | 17 | 1.8 | 29 | 11 | 0.3 |
| 78 | 331 | 1 | 0.1 | 18 | 0 | 0 |
| | | | | | | |
| 17 | 73 | 1 | 0.2 | 2 | 0 | 0 |
| 37 | 157 | 0 | 0.9 | 6 | 3 | 0 |
| 218 | 912 | 14 | 1.4 | 8 | 16 | 0.6 |
| 154 | 650 | 5 | 0.6 | 10 | 20 | 0.6 |
| 273 | 1137 | 20 | 2.9 | 10 | 14 | 0.7 |
| 133 | 557 | 8 | 2 | 7 | 9 | 0.3 |
| 112 | 469 | 5 | 1.6 | 8 | 9 | 0.4 |
| 17 | 71 | 1 | 0.5 | 2 | 0 | 0 |
| 201 | 838 | 9 | 3.1 | 15 | 15 | 0.9 |
| 498 | 2103 | 24 | 6.9 | 43 | 32 | Trace |
| 147 | 608 | 14 | 2.5 | 5 | 1 | Trace |

## FISH PRODUCTS AND DISHES

| | AVERAGE PORTION g |
|---|---|
| Roe, cod, hard, coated in batter, fried | 160 |
| Roe, cod, hard, fried | 116 |
| Roe, herring, soft, fried | 85 |
| Salmon en croûte, shop bought | 100 |
| Taramasalata | 45 |
| Tuna pâté | 40 |

## SEAFOOD AND SHELLFISH

| | |
|---|---|
| Cockles, boiled | 25 |
| Cockles, bottled in vinegar | 25 |
| Crab, boiled, dressed with shell | 130 |
| Crab, canned in brine | 40 |
| Lobster, boiled, dressed with shell | 250 |
| Mussels, boiled and shelled | 40 |
| Mussels, canned or bottled without shells | 40 |
| Oysters, uncooked and shelled | 120 |
| Prawns, boiled and shelled | 60 |
| Scallops, steamed and shelled | 70 |
| Squid, in batter, fried | 120 |
| Whelks, boiled and shelled | 30 |
| Winkles, boiled and shelled | 30 |

## SEAFOOD PRODUCTS AND DISHES

| | |
|---|---|
| Crabsticks | 100 |
| Scampi, in breadcrumbs, frozen, fried | 170 |
| Seafood cocktail | 88 |
| Seafood pasta, shop bought | 290 |

Unless otherwise stated, values for bottled and canned seafood are for drained weights. Dishes are homemade unless otherwise stated.

| ENERGY kcal | ENERGY kJ | FAT g | SATURATED FAT g | PROTEIN g | CARBOHYDRATE g | FIBRE g |
|---|---|---|---|---|---|---|
| 302 | 1264 | 19 | 2.6 | 20 | 14 | 0.3 |
| 234 | 979 | 14 | 1.9 | 24 | 3 | 0.1 |
| 225 | 941 | 13 | 2.2 | 22 | 4 | 0.2 |
| 288 | 1202 | 19 | 3.1 | 12 | 18 | 0.3 |
| 227 | 935 | 24 | 1.8 | 1 | 2 | Trace |
| 94 | 393 | 7 | 3.1 | 7 | 0 | Trace |
| | | | | | | |
| 13 | 57 | 1 | 0.1 | 3 | Trace | 0 |
| 15 | 63 | 1 | 0.1 | 3 | Trace | 0 |
| 166 | 696 | 7 | 0.9 | 25 | Trace | 0 |
| 31 | 130 | 0 | 0 | 7 | Trace | 0 |
| 258 | 1088 | 4 | 0.5 | 55 | Trace | 0 |
| 42 | 176 | 1 | 0.2 | 7 | 1 | 0 |
| 39 | 166 | 1 | 0.2 | 7 | 1 | 0 |
| 78 | 330 | 2 | 0.2 | 13 | 3 | 0 |
| 59 | 251 | 1 | 0.1 | 14 | 0 | 0 |
| 83 | 351 | 1 | 0.3 | 16 | 2 | Trace |
| 234 | 978 | 12 | 2.5 | 14 | 19 | 0.6 |
| 27 | 113 | 1 | 0.1 | 6 | Trace | 0 |
| 22 | 92 | 1 | 0.1 | 5 | Trace | 0 |
| | | | | | | |
| 68 | 290 | 0 | 0 | 10 | 7 | 0 |
| 403 | 1685 | 23 | 2.4 | 16 | 35 | 0 |
| 77 | 325 | 1 | 0.3 | 14 | 3 | 0 |
| 319 | 1334 | 14 | 8.1 | 26 | 22 | 1.2 |

FISH & SEAFOOD

| BURGER KING | AVERAGE PORTION g |
|---|---|
| Bacon and Egg Sandwich | 139 |
| Big King® | 202 |
| BK Chicken Flamer | 162 |
| BK Spicy Beanburger | 239 |
| Cajun Chicken Deli Wrap | 208 |
| Cheeseburger | 129 |
| Chicken Caesar Deli Wrap | 208 |
| Chicken Royale | 210 |
| Chicken Royale Club | 241 |
| Chicken Whopper | 260 |
| Chicken Whopper Junior | 159 |
| Chicken Whopper Lite | 161 |
| Double Cheeseburger | 185 |
| Double Cheeseburger with Bacon | 195 |
| Hamburger | 117 |
| Hash Browns, large | 102 |
| Hash Browns, medium | 68 |
| Kids Cheeseburger | 120 |
| Kids Hamburger | 107 |
| Kids Veggie Burger | 165 |
| King Fries, large | 142 |
| King Fries, regular | 116 |
| King Fries, small | 74 |
| Onion Rings, large | 120 |
| Onion Rings, regular | 90 |
| Sausage and Egg Sandwich | 160 |
| Sausage, Bacon and Egg Sandwich | 182 |
| Veggie Burger | 223 |
| Whopper® | 267 |
| Whopper Junior | 151 |
| Whopper Junior with Cheese | 163 |
| Whopper with Cheese | 292 |
| XL Double Whopper | 348 |
| XL Double Whopper with Cheese | 373 |

Information copyright © Burger King

| ENERGY kcal | ENERGY kJ | FAT g | SATURATED FAT g | PROTEIN g | CARBOHYDRATE g | FIBRE g |
|---|---|---|---|---|---|---|
| 296 | 1153 | 13 | 3.7 | 15 | 30 | 2.7 |
| 540 | 2163 | 31.3 | 12.8 | 33.3 | 30.3 | 2.2 |
| 308 | 1295 | 12 | 2.3 | 20 | 30 | 3.1 |
| 505 | 2112 | 20 | 5.8 | 19 | 63 | 9.3 |
| 511 | 2146 | 27.5 | 3.9 | 18 | 48 | 3.1 |
| 331 | 1289 | 14 | 6.4 | 20 | 30 | 1.8 |
| 835 | 1682 | 25.5 | 3.9 | 18.3 | 45.5 | 3.0 |
| 638 | 2696 | 40 | 1.4 | 25 | 47 | 4.9 |
| 668 | 2823 | 42.1 | 2.4 | 26.9 | 47.7 | 5.3 |
| 548 | 2300 | 23.4 | 1.3 | 39.4 | 45 | 2.5 |
| 339 | 1425 | 13.9 | 0.7 | 24.3 | 29.3 | 1.7 |
| 289 | 1223 | 7.5 | 1.1 | 25 | 29.9 | 1.7 |
| 492 | 1961 | 26 | 12.4 | 33 | 30 | 2.1 |
| 509 | 2034 | 28.3 | 13.3 | 37.4 | 30.7 | 2.1 |
| 290 | 1120 | 11 | 4.2 | 17 | 30 | 1.8 |
| 318 | 1330 | 19.7 | 4.4 | 2.2 | 33.0 | 3.8 |
| 212 | 887 | 13 | 2.9 | 2 | 22 | 2.6 |
| 328 | 1276 | 14 | 6.4 | 19.4 | 29.9 | 1.7 |
| 287 | 1107 | 10.6 | 4.2 | 17 | 29.7 | 1.7 |
| 359 | 1512 | 11.1 | 1.1 | 11.9 | 52.8 | 7.1 |
| 490 | 2047 | 19.6 | 3.4 | 3.7 | 52.7 | 3.6 |
| 400 | 1672 | 16 | 2.8 | 3 | 43 | 2.9 |
| 259 | 1081 | 10.2 | 1.8 | 1.9 | 32.3 | 1.9 |
| 348 | 1458 | 16.7 | 1.9 | 5.8 | 43.7 | 4.6 |
| 261 | 1094 | 13 | 1.4 | 4 | 33 | 3.4 |
| 375 | 1481 | 19 | 5.5 | 20 | 32 | 3 |
| 430 | 1712 | 23.1 | 7.4 | 24.1 | 31.8 | 3.1 |
| 432 | 1818 | 17 | 3.5 | 15 | 55 | 7.6 |
| 646 | 2583 | 38 | 8.1 | 31 | 48 | 3.6 |
| 372 | 1475 | 19.6 | 4.4 | 17.4 | 30.6 | 2.1 |
| 413 | 1644 | 23 | 6.6 | 19.8 | 30.7 | 2.1 |
| 728 | 2921 | 44.7 | 12.5 | 35.4 | 47.9 | 3.6 |
| 873 | 3531 | 53.9 | 15.2 | 51.6 | 47.6 | 4.2 |
| 955 | 3869 | 60.7 | 19.6 | 56.4 | 47.9 | 4.2 |

FASTFOODS

| KENTUCKY FRIED CHICKEN | AVERAGE PORTION g |
|---|---|
| BBQ Beans, large | 320 |
| BBQ Beans, regular | 125 |
| Cheese slice | 59 |
| Chicken drumstick (1) | 72.5 |
| Chicken Fillet Burger (with mayonnaise) | 213.7 |
| Chicken Fillet Burger (without mayonnaise) | 213.7 |
| Chicken Fillet Tower | 247.9 |
| Chicken Rib | 110.61 |
| Chicken Thigh | 103.6 |
| Chicken Wings | 71.07 |
| Coleslaw, large | 200 |
| Coleslaw, regular | 99.32 |
| Corn cobette (with butter) | 65 |
| Corn cobette (without butter) | 65 |
| Crispy Strips (1) | 36.75 |
| Fried chicken (2 pieces) | 372 |
| Fries, large | 149.22 |
| Fries, regular | 114.8 |
| Popcorn | 100 |
| Popcorn chicken, large | 218 |
| Popcorn chicken, regular | 147 |
| Twister (with pepper mayonnaise) | 224.8 |
| Twister (without pepper mayonnaise) | 211.3 |
| Zinger Burger | 185.4 |
| Zinger Burger with cheese slice | 198.9 |
| Zinger Tower Burger (with mayonnaise) | 256.1 |
| Zinger Tower Burger (without mayonnaise) | 249.6 |

| ENERGY kcal | ENERGY kJ | FAT g | SATURATED FAT g | PROTEIN g | CARBOHYDRATE g | FIBRE g |
|---|---|---|---|---|---|---|
| 294.4 | 1231.8 | 1.12 | 0.224 | 13.92 | 56.96 | 9.21 |
| 115 | 481.17 | 0.42 | 0.084 | 5.22 | 21.36 | 4.14 |
| 194.1 | 807 | 15.39 | 10.66 | 11.21 | 1.062 | 0 |
| 185 | 775 | 11.25 | 1.91 | 13.96 | 7.17 | 0.8 |
| | | | | | | |
| 470.85 | 1976.02 | 19.6 | 3.06 | 31.99 | 41.52 | 3.38 |
| | | | | | | |
| 408.94 | 1716 | 17.06 | 2.64 | 27.78 | 36.07 | 2.94 |
| 574.3 | 2406 | 27.82 | 5.6 | 27.78 | 49.02 | 3.6 |
| 292 | 1222 | 17.21 | 2.38 | 24.13 | 10.02 | 1.16 |
| 288 | 1199 | 20.35 | 4.27 | 19.92 | 5.8 | 0.87 |
| 574.3 | 2406 | 27.82 | 5.6 | 27.78 | 49.02 | 3.6 |
| 294 | 1212 | 26.9 | 1.6 | 1.86 | 10.92 | 2.66 |
| 146 | 606 | 13.45 | 0.8 | 0.93 | 5.46 | 1.33 |
| 68.68 | 290 | 1.69 | 0.76 | 2.13 | 11.27 | 1.40 |
| 79.7 | 336.96 | 1.5 | 0 | 2.66 | 14.77 | 3.05 |
| 113.23 | 472.92 | 6.37 | 0.98 | 7.63 | 6.11 | 0.61 |
| 1551 | 2305.43 | 23 | 3.8 | 28 | 14 | 0.8 |
| 382 | 1600 | 19.22 | 4.46 | 4.95 | 47.38 | 3.97 |
| 294 | 1232 | 14.78 | 3.43 | 3.81 | 36.44 | 3.06 |
| 264.5 | 1104.75 | 16.075 | 2.35 | 17.25 | 12.75 | 1.025 |
| 573.97 | 2397.31 | 35 | 4.95 | 37.5 | 27.62 | 1.06 |
| 388.82 | 1623.98 | 24 | 3.35 | 25.4 | 18.71 | 0.72 |
| 541.37 | 2262 | 30.02 | 6.26 | 23.5 | 43.88 | 4.14 |
| 499.51 | 2090 | 29.07 | 6.07 | 22.77 | 42.49 | 4.00 |
| 440 | 1847 | 19.33 | 2.89 | 25.49 | 41.05 | 2.56 |
| 490.60 | 2055.92 | 19.6 | 5.37 | 26.11 | 41.82 | 2.59 |
| | | | | | | |
| 607.29 | 2546 | 31.24 | 6.65 | 30.99 | 50.62 | 3.17 |
| | | | | | | |
| 555.51 | 2324.31 | 25.5 | 6.81 | 31.68 | 51.73 | 3.25 |

## INDIAN DISHES

| | AVERAGE PORTION g |
|---|---|
| Chicken biryani | 400 |
| Chicken dhansak | 350 |
| Chicken dupiaza | 350 |
| Chicken jalfrezi | 350 |
| Chicken korma | 350 |
| Chicken tikka | 350 |
| Chicken tikka masala | 350 |
| Lamb balti | 350 |
| Lamb rogan josh | 350 |
| Meat samosas | 70 |
| Poppadoms | 70 |
| Prawn bhuna | 400 |
| Prawn madras | 350 |
| Vegetable balti | 350 |
| Vegetable biryani | 350 |

## ORIENTAL DISHES

| | |
|---|---|
| Aromatic crispy duck | 125 |
| Chicken chop suey | 450 |
| Chicken chow mein | 350 |
| Chicken fried rice | 350 |
| Chicken satay | 170 |
| Chicken with cashew nuts | 360 |
| Egg fried rice | 270 |
| Green chicken curry | 350 |
| Meat spring roll | 55 |
| Pancakes | 70 |
| Prawn crackers | 70 |
| Sesame prawn toasts | 70 |
| Spare ribs | 340 |
| Stir-fried beef with green peppers in black bean sauce | 360 |
| Stir-fried Thai vegetable curry | 350 |

| ENERGY kcals | ENERGY kJ | FAT g | SATURATED FAT g | PROTEIN g | CARBOHYDRATE g | FIBRE g |
|---|---|---|---|---|---|---|
| 651 | 2144 | 30 | 8.0 | 34 | 66 | 4.4 |
| 503 | 1509 | 30 | 6.0 | 40 | 21 | 6.7 |
| 397 | 1168 | 25 | 4.9 | 40 | 4 | 6.3 |
| 416 | 1203 | 27 | 5.3 | 34 | 11 | 7.0 |
| 668 | 1753 | 51 | 20.0 | 44 | 8 | 7.0 |
| 421 | 1470 | 15 | 5.6 | 71 | Trace | 1.0 |
| 551 | 1488 | 40 | 13.7 | 47 | Trace | 7.7 |
| 534 | 1518 | 35 | 8.8 | 43 | 11 | 6.7 |
| 510 | 1422 | 35 | 9.8 | 43 | 6 | 3.1 |
| 191 | 553 | 12 | 3.2 | 8 | 13 | 1.5 |
| 351 | 916 | 27 | 5.6 | 8 | 20 | 4.1 |
| 363 | 802 | 35 | 4.0 | 6 | 7 | 7.6 |
| 390 | 1042 | 29 | 3.5 | 27 | 6 | 7.0 |
| 373 | 983 | 28 | 5.3 | 8 | 23 | 7.7 |
| 467 | 1468 | 25 | 4.9 | 10 | 55 | 6.0 |
| | | | | | | |
| 412 | 1107 | 30 | 9.1 | 35 | 15 | 1.1 |
| 363 | 1095 | 21 | 3.6 | 37 | 7 | 5.4 |
| 516 | 1662 | 25 | 4.2 | 30 | 46 | 3.9 |
| 562 | 1948 | 21 | 3.5 | 23 | 75 | 0.0 |
| 324 | 1006 | 18 | 4.9 | 37 | 5 | 3.7 |
| 470 | 1331 | 31 | 5.4 | 38 | 10 | 0.0 |
| 491 | 1809 | 13 | 1.6 | 12 | 87 | 2.2 |
| 417 | 1125 | 30 | 18.2 | 31 | 5 | 8.4 |
| 133 | 374 | 9 | 2.1 | 4 | 10 | 1.0 |
| 213 | 790 | 6 | Trace | 6 | 37 | 0.0 |
| 386 | 1061 | 27 | 2.6 | 0 | 37 | 0.8 |
| 268 | 699 | 21 | 2.7 | 9 | 12 | 1.3 |
| 873 | 2358 | 64 | 10.2 | 75 | 7 | 1.0 |
| | | | | | | |
| 373 | 1158 | 20 | 5.0 | 38 | 11 | 6.5 |
| 351 | 882 | 29 | 13.7 | 13 | 11 | 9.1 |

## ORIENTAL DISHES

| | AVERAGE PORTION g |
|---|---|
| Stir-fried vegetables | 340 |
| Sweet and sour chicken | 300 |
| Sweet and sour pork, battered | 300 |
| Szechuan prawns with vegetables | 350 |

## BURGERS AND HOTDOGS

| | |
|---|---|
| Cheeseburger, large, double | 258 |
| Cheeseburger, large, single | 219 |
| Cheeseburger, regular, double | 228 |
| Cheeseburger, triple, plain | 304 |
| Hamburger, large, double | 226 |
| Hamburger, large, single, with seasoning and sauce | 172 |
| Hamburger, large, triple patty, seasoning and sauce | 259 |
| Hamburger, regular, double, plain | 176 |
| Hamburger, regular, double, with seasoning and sauce | 215 |
| Hamburger, regular, single, plain | 90 |
| Hamburger, regular, single, with seasoning and sauce | 106 |

## MEXICAN DISHES

| | |
|---|---|
| Burrito, beans | 217 |
| Burrito, beans and cheese | 186 |
| Burrito, beans and chilli peppers | 204 |
| Burrito, beans and meat | 231 |
| Burrito, beans, cheese and beef | 203 |
| Burrito, beef | 220 |
| Burrito, beef and chilli peppers | 201 |
| Burrito, beef, cheese and chilli peppers | 304 |
| Chimichanga, beef | 174 |

Unless otherwise specified, burgers include garnish, seasonings and sauce.

| ENERGY kcals | ENERGY kJ | FAT g | SATURATED FAT g | PROTEIN g | CARBOHYDRATE g | FIBRE g |
|---|---|---|---|---|---|---|
| 177 | 455 | 14 | 2.4 | 6 | 7 | 6.1 |
| 575 | 1810 | 30 | 3.9 | 23 | 57 | 1.8 |
| 705 | 2115 | 42 | 6.9 | 23 | 63 | 3.0 |
| 297 | 912 | 16 | 1.8 | 27 | 11 | 4.9 |
| 704 | 2946 | 44 | 17.7 | 38 | 40 | 2.1 |
| 563 | 2354 | 33 | 15 | 28 | 38 | 2.1 |
| 650 | 2718 | 35 | 12.8 | 30 | 53 | 2.1 |
| 796 | 3332 | 51 | 21.7 | 56 | 27 | 2.1 |
| 540 | 2260 | 27 | 10.5 | 34 | 40 | 2.1 |
| 427 | 1785 | 21 | 7.9 | 23 | 37 | 2.1 |
| 692 | 2893 | 41 | 15.9 | 50 | 29 | 2.1 |
| 544 | 2276 | 28 | 10.4 | 30 | 43 | 2 |
| 576 | 2410 | 32 | 12 | 32 | 39 | 2.1 |
| 274 | 1148 | 12 | 4.1 | 12 | 31 | 2 |
| 272 | 1140 | 10 | 3.6 | 12 | 34 | 2.3 |
| 447 | 1871 | 13 | 6.9 | 14 | 71 | 1.5 |
| 378 | 1579 | 12 | 6.8 | 15 | 55 | 1.5 |
| 412 | 1724 | 15 | 7.6 | 16 | 58 | 1.5 |
| 508 | 2125 | 18 | 8.3 | 22 | 66 | 1.5 |
| 331 | 1384 | 13 | 7.1 | 15 | 40 | 1.5 |
| 524 | 2191 | 21 | 10.5 | 27 | 59 | 1.5 |
| 426 | 1783 | 17 | 8 | 22 | 49 | 1.5 |
| 632 | 2645 | 25 | 10.4 | 41 | 64 | 1.5 |
| 425 | 1777 | 20 | 8.5 | 20 | 43 | 1.5 |

## MEXICAN DISHES

| | AVERAGE PORTION g |
|---|---|
| Chimichanga, beef and cheese | 183 |
| Chimichanga, beef and chilli peppers | 190 |
| Chimichanga, beef, cheese and chilli peppers | 180 |
| Enchilada, cheese | 163 |
| Enchilada, cheese and beef | 192 |
| Enchilada, vegetable | 360 |
| Fajita, chicken, meat only | 170 |
| Nachos, cheese | 113 |
| Nachos, cheese and jalapeno peppers | 204 |
| Nachos, cheese, beans, ground beef and peppers | 255 |

## PIZZA

| | |
|---|---|
| Pizza, cheese and tomato, deep pan, shop bought | 220 |
| Pizza, cheese and tomato, deep pan | 220 |
| Pizza, cheese and tomato, French bread, frozen, shop bought | 200 |
| Pizza, cheese and tomato, frozen, shop bought | 200 |
| Pizza, cheese and tomato, thin base | 116 |
| Pizza, chicken, deep pan, shop bought | 230 |
| Pizza, fish topped, deep pan | 230 |
| Pizza, fish topped, thin base | 150 |
| Pizza, ham and pineapple, shop bought | 200 |
| Pizza, meat topped, deep pan | 230 |
| Pizza, meat topped, frozen, shop bought | 200 |
| Pizza, meat topped, thin base | 150 |
| Pizza, meat, deep pan, shop bought | 230 |
| Pizza, vegetable topped, deep pan | 290 |
| Pizza, vegetable topped, thin base | 150 |

Unless otherwise specified, pizzas are takeaway.

| ENERGY kcals | ENERGY kJ | FAT g | SATURATED FAT g | PROTEIN g | CARBOHYDRATE g | FIBRE g |
|---|---|---|---|---|---|---|
| 443 | 1854 | 23 | 11.2 | 20 | 39 | 1.5 |
| 424 | 1773 | 19 | 8.3 | 18 | 46 | 1.5 |
| | | | | | | |
| 364 | 1521 | 18 | 8.4 | 15 | 38 | 1.5 |
| 319 | 1337 | 19 | 10.6 | 10 | 29 | 1 |
| 323 | 1350 | 18 | 9 | 12 | 30 | 1 |
| 525 | 1690 | 26 | 7.6 | 23 | 54 | 7.6 |
| 213 | 676 | 11 | 3.6 | 29 | 1 | 1.7 |
| 438 | 1208 | 31 | 11.6 | 18 | 24 | 3.4 |
| 608 | 2544 | 34 | 14 | 17 | 60 | 2 |
| | | | | | | |
| 569 | 2379 | 31 | 12.5 | 20 | 56 | 2 |
| | | | | | | |
| 471 | 1987 | 15 | 7.7 | 24 | 64 | 4.8 |
| 547 | 2310 | 16 | 11.4 | 27 | 77 | 4.8 |
| | | | | | | |
| 461 | 1942 | 16 | 6.6 | 21 | 63 | 3.8 |
| | | | | | | |
| 475 | 2002 | 18 | 9 | 23 | 60 | 3.8 |
| 322 | 1355 | 12 | 9.3 | 17 | 39 | 2.2 |
| 565 | 2382 | 19 | 7.8 | 31 | 72 | 4.8 |
| 507 | 2138 | 16 | 6.2 | 30 | 64 | 4.6 |
| 343 | 1446 | 12 | 9.2 | 20 | 41 | 2.8 |
| 521 | 2196 | 17 | 6.8 | 27 | 69 | 4.8 |
| 557 | 2345 | 21 | 14 | 30 | 67 | 4.6 |
| | | | | | | |
| 496 | 2087 | 19 | 7.6 | 23 | 61 | 3.8 |
| 391 | 1642 | 18 | 7.5 | 21 | 39 | 2.8 |
| 624 | 2624 | 25 | 9.7 | 32 | 73 | 4.8 |
| 621 | 2624 | 18 | 7.8 | 32 | 88 | 4.9 |
| 332 | 1398 | 11 | 4.1 | 16 | 44 | 2.8 |

TAKEAWAY
DISHES **75**

| RICE, PASTA AND NOODLES | AVERAGE PORTION g |
|---|---|
| Brown rice, boiled | 180 |
| Macaroni, boiled | 230 |
| Macaroni, wholemeal, boiled | 230 |
| Noodles, egg, boiled | 230 |
| Noodles, boiled | 230 |
| Noodles, fried | 230 |
| Red rice, boiled | 230 |
| Savoury rice, cooked | 180 |
| Spaghetti, boiled | 220 |
| Spaghetti, wholemeal, boiled | 230 |
| White rice, easy cook, boiled | 180 |
| White rice, fried in lard/dripping | 300 |
| White rice, glutinous, boiled | 230 |
| White rice, polished, boiled | 230 |

## RICE AND PASTA DISHES

| | |
|---|---|
| Cannelloni, meat, shop bought | 260 |
| Cannelloni, spinach | 340 |
| Cannelloni, vegetable | 340 |
| Chicken risotto | 340 |
| Lasagne, meat, shop bought | 420 |
| Lasagne, spinach | 420 |
| Lasagne, spinach, wholemeal | 420 |
| Lasagne, vegetable | 420 |
| Lasagne, vegetable, wholemeal | 420 |
| Pasta with ham and mushroom sauce | 235 |
| Pasta with meat and tomato sauce | 235 |
| Peppers, stuffed with rice | 175 |
| Pilau, mushroom | 180 |
| Pilau, vegetable | 180 |
| Ravioli, stuffed with cheese, tomato and herbs, shop bought | 250 |

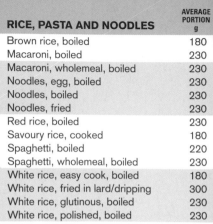

Unless otherwise stated, all dishes are homemade.

| ENERGY kcal | ENERGY kJ | FAT g | SATURATED FAT g | PROTEIN g | CARBOHYDRATE g | FIBRE g |
|---|---|---|---|---|---|---|
| 254 | 1075 | 2 | 0.5 | 5 | 58 | 1.4 |
| 198 | 840 | 1 | 0.2 | 7 | 43 | 2.1 |
| 198 | 840 | 1 | 0.2 | 7 | 43 | 6.4 |
| 143 | 607 | 1 | 0.2 | 5 | 30 | 1.4 |
| 143 | 607 | 1 | 0.2 | 6 | 30 | 1.6 |
| 352 | 1467 | 26 | 1 | 4 | 26 | 1.2 |
| 184 | 784 | 1 | 0.2 | 4 | 43 | 1.4 |
| 256 | 1078 | 6 | 2 | 5 | 47 | 2.5 |
| 229 | 972 | 2 | 0.2 | 8 | 49 | 2.6 |
| 260 | 1116 | 2 | 0.2 | 11 | 53 | 8.1 |
| 248 | 1057 | 2 | 0.5 | 5 | 56 | 0.2 |
| 393 | 1662 | 10 | 4.2 | 7 | 75 | 1.8 |
| 150 | 633 | 1 | 0.2 | 4 | 34 | 0.5 |
| 283 | 1201 | 1 | 0.2 | 5 | 68 | 0.5 |
| | | | | | | |
| 315 | 1326 | 13 | 5.2 | 17 | 35 | 3.1 |
| 449 | 1880 | 26 | 7.8 | 15 | 43 | 2.7 |
| 493 | 2067 | 31 | 11.6 | 15 | 43 | 2.4 |
| 546 | 2310 | 10 | 4.5 | 31 | 84 | Trace |
| 601 | 2533 | 26 | 11.8 | 31 | 66 | 2.9 |
| 365 | 1541 | 13 | 5.5 | 15 | 53 | 4.6 |
| 391 | 1659 | 13 | 5.5 | 18 | 55 | 9.7 |
| 428 | 1810 | 18 | 9.2 | 17 | 52 | 4.2 |
| 445 | 1877 | 19 | 9.2 | 20 | 52 | 8.8 |
| 284 | 1194 | 14 | 8.2 | 13 | 27 | 2.1 |
| 263 | 1102 | 10 | 4 | 16 | 30 | 2 |
| 149 | 630 | 4 | 0.7 | 3 | 27 | 2.3 |
| 248 | 1048 | 8 | 4.5 | 4 | 43 | 0.7 |
| 248 | 1053 | 8 | 4.3 | 5 | 43 | 1 |
| 304 | 1267 | 13 | 7.9 | 17 | 30 | 0.6 |

RICE, PASTA
& NOODLES

## RICE AND PASTA DISHES

| | AVERAGE PORTION g |
|---|---|
| Ravioli, stuffed with meat and vegetables, shop bought | 250 |
| Rice and blackeye beans | 200 |
| Rice and blackeye beans, brown rice | 200 |
| Risotto, chicken | 340 |
| Risotto, vegetable, brown rice | 290 |
| Risotto, vegetable | 290 |
| Spaghetti bolognese, shop bought | 400 |
| Tortellini, stuffed with cheese and ham, shop bought | 250 |
| Vine leaves, stuffed with rice | 80 |

Unless otherwise stated, all dishes are homemade.

| ENERGY kcal | ENERGY kJ | FAT g | SATURATED FAT g | PROTEIN g | CARBOHYDRATE g | FIBRE g |
|---|---|---|---|---|---|---|
| 324 | 1350 | 15 | 8.9 | 16 | 34 | 3.4 |
| 366 | 1556 | 7 | 3 | 12 | 68 | 2.8 |
| 350 | 1488 | 7 | 3 | 11 | 66 | 3.6 |
| 546 | 2310 | 10 | 4.5 | 31 | 84 | Trace |
| 415 | 1749 | 19 | 2.6 | 12 | 54 | 7 |
| 426 | 1798 | 19 | 2.9 | 12 | 56 | 6.4 |
| 432 | 1816 | 23 | 9.2 | 37 | 21 | 3.6 |
| 316 | 1318 | 9 | 6 | 16 | 44 | 1.4 |
| 210 | 875 | 14 | 2.1 | 2 | 19 | 1.0 |

| BREAD, CAKES, SCONES AND PASTRIES | AVERAGE PORTION g |
|---|---|
| Asian pastries | 40 |
| Banana loaf, homemade, no icing | 85 |
| Battenburg cake | 32 |
| Brioche | 45 |
| Brown bread, sliced | 36 |
| Brown rolls/baps | 48 |
| Burfi | 40 |
| Carrot cake, homemade, no icing | 85 |
| Cheese-topped rolls/baps, white | 85 |
| Chelsea buns | 78 |
| Cherry cake | 38 |
| Chinese flaky pastries | 40 |
| Chocolate cake | 40 |
| Chocolate cake, with butter icing | 65 |
| Chocolate fudge cake | 98 |
| Choux buns | 112 |
| Ciabatta, plain | 50 |
| Coconut cake | 40 |
| Cream horns | 60 |
| Crispie cakes | 31 |
| Croissants | 60 |
| Crumpets | 40 |
| Currant buns | 60 |
| Custard tarts, individual | 94 |
| Danish pastries | 110 |
| Doughnuts, custard-filled | 75 |
| Doughnuts, jam | 75 |
| Doughnuts, ring | 60 |
| Doughnuts, ring, iced | 75 |
| Eccles cake | 45 |
| Eclairs, fresh | 112 |
| Fancy iced cakes, individual | 30 |
| Focaccia, herb/garlic and coriander | 50 |
| French baguette, white | 40 |

| ENERGY kcal | ENERGY kJ | FAT g | SATURATED FAT g | PROTEIN g | CARBOHYDRATE g | FIBRE g |
|---|---|---|---|---|---|---|
| 215 | 897 | 16 | 8 | 3 | 17 | 0.8 |
| 230 | 968 | 9 | 5.6 | 4 | 35 | 1.5 |
| 118 | 496 | 6 | 1.5 | 2 | 16 | 0.4 |
| 144 | 607 | 4 | 2.8 | 4 | 24 | 1.0 |
| 75 | 317 | 1 | 0.2 | 3 | 15 | 1.3 |
| 113 | 482 | 2 | 0.3 | 5 | 22 | 1.8 |
| 117 | 487 | 8 | 4 | 5 | 7 | 0.8 |
| 349 | 1454 | 25 | 6.4 | 5 | 28 | 2.1 |
| 241 | 1016 | 7 | 3.4 | 9 | 38 | 1.2 |
| 285 | 1203 | 11 | 3.3 | 6 | 44 | 1.3 |
| 150 | 630 | 6 | 1.6 | 2 | 23 | 0.4 |
| 157 | 659 | 7 | 4 | 2 | 24 | 0.8 |
| 182 | 763 | 11 | 8.2 | 3 | 20 | 0.5 |
| 313 | 1306 | 19 | 14.3 | 4 | 33 | 0.8 |
| 351 | 1479 | 14 | 4.5 | 5 | 55 | 0.9 |
| 427 | 1766 | 36 | 19 | 6 | 20 | 0.8 |
| 135 | 574 | 2 | 0.3 | 5 | 26 | 1.2 |
| 174 | 726 | 10 | 2.6 | 3 | 20 | 1 |
| 261 | 1082 | 21 | 10 | 2 | 15 | 0.5 |
| 144 | 605 | 6 | 3.3 | 2 | 23 | 0.1 |
| 224 | 938 | 12 | 5.9 | 5 | 26 | 1.0 |
| 83 | 352 | 1 | 0.2 | 3 | 18 | 0.8 |
| 178 | 750 | 5 | 2 | 5 | 32 | 1.6 |
| 260 | 1091 | 14 | 5.3 | 6 | 30 | 1.1 |
| 411 | 1728 | 16 | 6.2 | 6 | 56 | 1.8 |
| 269 | 1125 | 14 | 10.4 | 5 | 32 | 1.6 |
| 252 | 1061 | 11 | 3.2 | 4 | 37 | 1.6 |
| 238 | 997 | 13 | 3.8 | 4 | 28 | 1.4 |
| 287 | 1208 | 13 | 3.8 | 4 | 41 | 1.4 |
| 214 | 896 | 12 | 4.5 | 2 | 27 | 0.7 |
| 418 | 1746 | 27 | 14.3 | 5 | 42 | 0.6 |
| 122 | 515 | 3 | 2.8 | 1 | 21 | 0.4 |
| 147 | 620 | 4 | 0.6 | 5 | 26 | 0.7 |
| 109 | 465 | 1 | 0.1 | 4 | 24 | 1.0 |

BREAD, CAKES,
SCONES &
PASTRIES **81**

## BREAD, CAKES, SCONES AND PASTRIES

| | AVERAGE PORTION g |
|---|---|
| French baguette, white, part baked | 40 |
| French baton, granary | 40 |
| French stick/flute, white | 40 |
| Fruit buns, white, not iced | 78 |
| Fruit cake, plain | 60 |
| Fruit cake, rich | 70 |
| Fruit cake, rich, iced | 70 |
| Fruit cake, wholemeal | 90 |
| Garlic bread | 20 |
| Gingerbread | 50 |
| Granary bread, sliced | 36 |
| Granary rolls | 56 |
| Greek pastries | 100 |
| Gulab jamen/gulab jambu | 40 |
| Hot cross buns | 50 |
| Jam tarts | 34 |
| Jam tarts, wholemeal | 34 |
| Jellabi | 40 |
| Madeira | 40 |
| Malt loaf, fruit | 35 |
| Milk bread, white | 15 |
| Mince pies, individual | 55 |
| Muffins, English, white | 68 |
| Muffins, English, white, toasted | 68 |
| Naan bread, garlic and coriander/plain | 160 |
| Pitta bread, white | 75 |
| Pumpernickel bread | 33 |
| Rock cakes | 29 |
| Scones, cheese | 48 |
| Scones, fruit | 48 |
| Scones, plain | 48 |
| Scones, potato | 57 |
| Scones, wholemeal | 50 |
| Scones, wholemeal, fruit | 50 |

| ENERGY kcal | ENERGY kJ | FAT g | SATURATED FAT g | PROTEIN g | CARBOHYDRATE g | FIBRE g |
|---|---|---|---|---|---|---|
| 108 | 458 | 1 | 0.1 | 4 | 23 | 1.0 |
| 110 | 467 | 1 | 0.1 | 4 | 22 | 1.0 |
| 101 | 431 | 1 | 0.1 | 4 | 21 | 1.0 |
| 218 | 924 | 4 | 1.5 | 6 | 41 | 1.7 |
| 212 | 894 | 9 | 3.5 | 3 | 35 | 1.6 |
| 239 | 1007 | 8 | 2.4 | 3 | 42 | 1.2 |
| 249 | 1053 | 8 | 1.8 | 3 | 44 | 1.2 |
| 327 | 1373 | 14 | 4.3 | 5 | 48 | 2.2 |
| 73 | 306 | 4 | 1.9 | 2 | 9 | 1.0 |
| 190 | 799 | 6 | 1.9 | 3 | 32 | 0.6 |
| 87 | 369 | 1 | 0.3 | 4 | 18 | 1.3 |
| 133 | 565 | 2 | 0.3 | 6 | 24 | 2.0 |
| 322 | 1349 | 17 | 9 | 5 | 40 | 0.8 |
| 143 | 602 | 6 | 3 | 3 | 21 | 0.1 |
| 155 | 657 | 3 | 1 | 4 | 29 | 0.9 |
| 125 | 527 | 5 | 1.6 | 1 | 22 | 0.4 |
| 125 | 528 | 5 | 1.6 | 1 | 20 | 1.2 |
| 145 | 611 | 5 | 3 | 2 | 24 | 0.5 |
| 157 | 661 | 6 | 3.5 | 2 | 23 | 0.4 |
| 18 | 76 | 1 | 0.2 | 3 | 22.7 | 0.9 |
| 36 | 153 | 1 | 0.2 | 1 | 7 | 0.3 |
| 233 | 975 | 11 | 4.1 | 2 | 32 | 1.2 |
| 152 | 644 | 1 | 0.3 | 7 | 30 | 1.3 |
| 177 | 753 | 2 | 0.3 | 8 | 35 | 1.3 |
| 456 | 1929 | 12 | 1.6 | 12 | 80 | 3.2 |
| 191 | 813 | 1 | 0.7 | 7 | 41 | 1.8 |
| 67 | 283 | 1 | 0.1 | 2 | 15 | 2.1 |
| 115 | 483 | 5 | 1 | 2 | 18 | 0.4 |
| 174 | 731 | 9 | 4.9 | 5 | 21 | 0.8 |
| 152 | 640 | 5 | 1.6 | 4 | 25 | 0.8 |
| 174 | 731 | 7 | 2.4 | 3 | 26 | 0.9 |
| 169 | 707 | 8 | 4.4 | 3 | 22 | 0.9 |
| 163 | 684 | 7 | 2.4 | 4 | 22 | 2.6 |
| 162 | 683 | 6 | 2 | 4 | 24 | 2.5 |

BREAD, CAKES,
SCONES &
PASTRIES **83**

| BREAD, CAKES, SCONES AND PASTRIES | AVERAGE PORTION g |
|---|---|
| Scotch pancakes | 31 |
| Slimmers white bread, sliced | 20 |
| Soda bread, brown | 130 |
| Sponge, fatless | 58 |
| Sponge, frozen | 60 |
| Sponge, jam-filled | 60 |
| Sponge, with butter icing | 60 |
| Strawberry tartlets | 54 |
| Swiss roll | 30 |
| Swiss rolls, chocolate, individual | 30 |
| Teacakes | 55 |
| Tortilla, soft | 160 |
| Vanilla slices | 113 |
| Waffles | 65 |
| Wheatgerm bread | 30 |
| White bread, crusty bloomer | 35 |
| White bread, farmhouse, large | 35 |
| White bread, farmhouse, small | 27 |
| White bread, premium | 36 |
| White bread, standard | 36 |
| White bread, standard, toasted | 36 |
| White rolls, crusty | 50 |
| White rolls, soft | 45 |
| Wholemeal bread | 38 |
| Wholemeal bread, toasted | 38 |
| Wholemeal rolls | 48 |

| ENERGY kcal | ENERGY kJ | FAT g | SATURATED FAT g | PROTEIN g | CARBOHYDRATE g | FIBRE g |
|---|---|---|---|---|---|---|
| 91 | 381 | 4 | 1.3 | 2 | 14 | 0.4 |
| 46 | 193 | 1 | 0.1 | 2 | 9 | 0.5 |
| 267 | 1132 | 4 | 1.0 | 11 | 50 | 4.9 |
| 171 | 722 | 4 | 1 | 6 | 31 | 0.5 |
| 190 | 795 | 10 | 3.1 | 2 | 24 | 0.4 |
| 181 | 768 | 3 | 1 | 3 | 39 | 1.1 |
| 294 | 1228 | 18 | 5.6 | 3 | 31 | 0.4 |
| 111 | 466 | 6 | 3.2 | 1 | 14 | 0.6 |
| 83 | 352 | 1 | 0.3 | 2 | 17 | 0.2 |
| 101 | 426 | 5 | 1.4 | 1 | 17 | 0.3 |
| 181 | 766 | 5 | 1.8 | 5 | 32 | 1.2 |
| 451 | 1903 | 14 | 2.9 | 12 | 73 | 3.0 |
| 373 | 1563 | 20 | 10.6 | 5 | 45 | 0.9 |
| 217 | 911 | 11 | 4.7 | 6 | 26 | 1 |
| 66 | 281 | 1 | 0.2 | 3 | 12 | 1.2 |
| 86 | 368 | 1 | 0.2 | 3 | 18 | 0.8 |
| 83 | 353 | 1 | 0.2 | 3 | 17 | 0.7 |
| 66 | 281 | 1 | 0.2 | 2 | 14 | 0.7 |
| 83 | 352 | 1 | 0.2 | 3 | 17 | 0.7 |
| 79 | 335 | 1 | 0.1 | 3 | 17 | 0.7 |
| 97 | 414 | 1 | 0.1 | 3 | 21 | 0.0 |
| 131 | 558 | 1 | 0.3 | 5 | 27 | 1.2 |
| 114 | 485 | 1 | 0.3 | 4 | 23 | 0.9 |
| 82 | 349 | 1 | 0.2 | 4 | 16 | 1.9 |
| 102 | 431 | 1 | 0.2 | 5 | 20 | 0.0 |
| 117 | 498 | 2 | 0.2 | 5 | 22 | 2.1 |

BREAD, CAKES,
SCONES &

| CHEESE | AVERAGE PORTION g |
|---|---|
| Brie, without rind | 40 |
| Camembert | 40 |
| Cheddar, English, white | 40 |
| Cheddar, half-fat (15% fat) | 40 |
| Cheddar, vegetarian | 40 |
| Cheese spread | 30 |
| Cheshire, white | 40 |
| Cottage (4% fat) | 40 |
| Cottage, low-fat (1.5–2% fat) | 40 |
| Danish Blue | 30 |
| Dolcelatte, without rind | 40 |
| Double Gloucester | 40 |
| Edam | 40 |
| Emmental | 40 |
| Fontina | 28 |
| Fromage frais, fruit | 100 |
| Fromage frais, fruit, virtually fat-free | 100 |
| Fromage frais, natural | 100 |
| Fromage frais, natural, virtually fat-free | 100 |
| Goats' milk | 55 |
| Gouda | 40 |
| Halloumi | 40 |
| Lancashire | 40 |
| Mascarpone | 55 |
| Monterey Jack | 28 |
| Mozzarella, fresh | 55 |
| Mozzarella, grated | 55 |
| Paneer | 40 |
| Parmesan, drums, freshly grated | 20 |
| Parmesan, wedges, freshly grated | 20 |
| Pecorino | 28 |
| Port Salut | 40 |
| Processed cheese, slices | 20 |
| Provolone | 28 |

Unless otherwise specified, generic cheeses are made with cows' milk.

| ENERGY kcal | ENERGY kJ | FAT g | SATURATED FAT g | PROTEIN g | CARBOHYDRATE g | FIBRE g |
|---|---|---|---|---|---|---|
| 144 | 596 | 12 | 7.3 | 8 | 2 | 0 |
| 116 | 482 | 9 | 6.0 | 9 | Trace | 0 |
| 166 | 690 | 14 | 8.7 | 10 | 0 | 0 |
| 109 | 456 | 6 | 4.3 | 13 | Trace | 0 |
| 156 | 647 | 13 | 8.3 | 10 | Trace | 0 |
| 81 | 335 | 7 | 4.7 | 3 | 2 | 0 |
| 152 | 630 | 13 | 8.5 | 9 | Trace | 0 |
| 36 | 149 | 2 | 0.9 | 5 | 0 | 0 |
| 28 | 118 | 1 | 0.4 | 5 | 0 | 0 |
| 103 | 425 | 9 | 5.7 | 6 | Trace | 0 |
| 158 | 652 | 14 | 8.7 | 7 | Trace | 0 |
| 165 | 684 | 14 | 9.3 | 10 | Trace | 0 |
| 136 | 566 | 10 | 6.3 | 11 | Trace | 0 |
| 160 | 663 | 12 | 8.2 | 12 | Trace | 0 |
| 110 | 462 | 9 | 5.4 | 7 | 0 | 0 |
| 135 | 566 | 5.6 | 0.0 | 5.2 | 16.9 | 0.4 |
| 50 | 211 | 0.2 | 0.0 | 6.7 | 5.6 | 0.4 |
| 113 | 468 | 8.0 | 5.6 | 6.0 | 4.4 | Trace |
| 48 | 205 | 0.1 | 0.0 | 7.5 | 4.6 | Trace |
| 174 | 722 | 14 | 9.8 | 12 | Trace | 0 |
| 151 | 625 | 12 | 8.1 | 10 | Trace | 0 |
| 124 | 516 | 9 | 6.6 | 10 | 0 | 0 |
| 153 | 633 | 13 | 8.4 | 10 | Trace | 0 |
| 230 | 949 | 24 | 16.2 | 3 | Trace | 0 |
| 107 | 443 | 30 | 5.4 | 25 | 0 | 0 |
| 141 | 587 | 11 | 7.6 | 10 | Trace | 0 |
| 164 | 680 | 12 | 8.1 | 14 | Trace | 0 |
| 130 | 539 | 10 | 6.2 | 10 | Trace | 0 |
| 97 | 403 | 7 | 4.6 | 9 | Trace | 0 |
| 82 | 343 | 6 | 3.9 | 7 | Trace | 0 |
| 110 | 459 | 8 | 4.8 | 1 | 1 | 0 |
| 133 | 554 | 10 | 7.2 | 10 | Trace | 0 |
| 59 | 244 | 5 | 2.8 | 4 | 1 | 0 |
| 99 | 417 | 8 | 4.8 | 7 | 1 | 0 |

## CHEESE

| | AVERAGE PORTION g |
|---|---|
| Red Leceister | 40 |
| Ricotta | 55 |
| Romano | 28 |
| Roquefort | 28 |
| Soft white spreadable, low-fat (<10%) | 30 |
| Soft white spreadable, medium-fat (15%) | 30 |
| Soft white spreadable, full-fat | 30 |
| St Paulin | 40 |
| Stilton, blue | 35 |
| Wensleydale | 40 |

## CREAM AND SUBSTITUTES

| | |
|---|---|
| Cream, clotted | 45 |
| Cream, double | 30 |
| Cream, half | 30 |
| Cream, single | 15 |
| Cream, soured | 30 |
| Cream, whipping | 30 |
| Cream, frozen, whipping | 30 |
| Cream, sterilised, canned | 45 |
| Cream, UHT, canned spray | 10 |
| Cream, UHT, half-fat | 15 |
| Cream, UHT, single | 15 |
| Cream, UHT, whipping | 30 |
| Crème fraîche | 50 |
| Crème fraîche, low-fat | 50 |
| Mock cream, double | 30 |
| Mock cream, single | 30 |
| Mock cream, whipping | 30 |

Unless otherwise specified, generic cheeses are made with cows' milk and cream is fresh.

| ENERGY kcal | ENERGY kJ | FAT g | SATURATED FAT g | PROTEIN g | CARBOHYDRATE g | FIBRE g |
|---|---|---|---|---|---|---|
| 161 | 667 | 13 | 8.9 | 10 | Trace | 0 |
| 79 | 329 | 6 | 3.8 | 5 | 1 | 0 |
| 110 | 459 | 8 | 4.8 | 1 | 1 | 0 |
| 105 | 438 | 9 | 5.4 | 6 | 1 | 0 |
| 43 | 182 | 2 | 1.7 | 4 | 1 | 0 |
| | | | | | | |
| 56 | 231 | 5 | 3.4 | 3 | Trace | 0 |
| 94 | 386 | 9 | 6.7 | 2 | Trace | 0 |
| 133 | 554 | 10 | 7.2 | 10 | Trace | 0 |
| 143 | 594 | 12 | 8.1 | 8 | Trace | 0 |
| 152 | 632 | 13 | 8.5 | 9 | Trace | 0 |
| | | | | | | |
| 264 | 1086 | 29 | 17.9 | 1 | 1 | 0 |
| 135 | 555 | 16 | 9 | 1 | 1 | 0 |
| 44 | 184 | 4 | 2.5 | 1 | 1 | 0 |
| 30 | 123 | 3 | 1.8 | 0 | 1 | 0 |
| 62 | 254 | 6 | 3.8 | 1 | 1 | 0 |
| 112 | 462 | 12 | 7.4 | 1 | 1 | 0 |
| 114 | 468 | 12 | 7.5 | 1 | 1 | 0 |
| 108 | 443 | 11 | 6.7 | 1 | 2 | 0 |
| 31 | 127 | 2 | 2 | 0 | 0 | 0 |
| 21 | 86 | 2 | 1.2 | 0 | 1 | 0 |
| 29 | 122 | 3 | 1.8 | 0 | 1 | 0 |
| 112 | 462 | 12 | 7.4 | 1 | 1 | 0 |
| 190 | 792 | 20 | 13.2 | 1.2 | 1.4 | 0 |
| 85 | 355 | 7.5 | 4.5 | 1.8 | 2.5 | 0 |
| 136 | 561 | 11 | 8.7 | 1 | 1 | 0 |
| 57 | 236 | 4 | 4.2 | 1 | 1 | 0 |
| 96 | 395 | 9 | 8.4 | 1 | 1 | 0 |

## EGGS

| | AVERAGE PORTION g |
|---|---|
| Battery, raw | 60 |
| Boiled | 50 |
| Duck, boiled and salted | 70 |
| Duck, raw | 75 |
| Egg yolk, raw | 18 |
| Free-range, raw | 60 |
| Fried in vegetable oil | 60 |
| Fried, without fat | 50 |
| Poached | 50 |
| Quail, raw | 40 |

## EGG DISHES

| | |
|---|---|
| Omelette, cheese | 150 |
| Omelette, plain (two-egg) | 120 |
| Omelette, Spanish (two-egg) | 150 |
| Scrambled, with milk (two-egg) | 120 |
| Scrambled, without milk (two-egg) | 100 |

## MILK AND MILK SUBSTITUTES

| | |
|---|---|
| Coffee whitener | 3 |
| Condensed milk, skimmed, sweetened | 15 |
| Condensed milk, whole, sweetened | 15 |
| Evaporated milk, reduced-fat | 15 |
| Evaporated milk, whole | 15 |
| Flavoured milk | 214 |
| Goats' milk, pasteurised | 146 |
| Semi-skimmed milk, pasteurised | 146 |
| Semi-skimmed milk, UHT | 146 |
| Sheep's milk | 146 |
| Skimmed milk, dried | 3 |
| Skimmed milk, dried, with vegetable fat | 3 |

Unless otherwise specified, figures are for one egg, chicken's eggs are medium-sized and milk is cows' milk.

| ENERGY kcal | ENERGY kJ | FAT g | SATURATED FAT g | PROTEIN g | CARBOHYDRATE g | FIBRE g |
|---|---|---|---|---|---|---|
| 88 | 367 | 6 | 1.9 | 8 | Trace | 0 |
| 74 | 306 | 5 | 1.5 | 6 | Trace | 0 |
| 139 | 575 | 11 | 2.7 | 10 | Trace | 0 |
| 122 | 510 | 9 | 2.2 | 11 | Trace | 0 |
| 61 | 252 | 5 | 1.6 | 3 | Trace | 0 |
| 86 | 358 | 7 | 1.7 | 7 | Trace | 0 |
| 107 | 447 | 8 | 2.4 | 8 | Trace | 0 |
| 87 | 363 | 6 | 1.8 | 8 | Trace | 0 |
| 74 | 306 | 5 | 1.5 | 6 | Trace | 0 |
| 60 | 252 | 4 | 1.2 | 5 | Trace | 0 |
| | | | | | | |
| 399 | 1659 | 18.3 | 34 | 24 | Trace | 0 |
| 229 | 950 | 8.9 | 20 | 13 | Trace | 0 |
| 180 | 752 | 2.4 | 12 | 9 | 9 | 2.1 |
| 296 | 1230 | 13.9 | 27 | 13 | 1 | 0 |
| 160 | 664 | 3.3 | 12 | 14 | Trace | 0 |
| | | | | | | |
| 16 | 68 | 1 | 1 | 0 | 2 | 0 |
| 40 | 171 | 0 | 0 | 2 | 9 | 0 |
| 50 | 211 | 2 | 0.9 | 1 | 8 | 0 |
| 18 | 77 | 1 | 0.2 | 1 | 2 | 0 |
| 23 | 94 | 1 | 0.9 | 1 | 1 | 0 |
| 146 | 614 | 3 | 1.9 | 8 | 23 | 0 |
| 88 | 369 | 5 | 3.4 | 5 | 6 | 0 |
| 67 | 285 | 2 | 1.5 | 5 | 7 | 0 |
| 67 | 283 | 2 | 1.6 | 5 | 7 | 0 |
| 139 | 578 | 8 | 5.5 | 8 | 7 | 0 |
| 10 | 44 | 0 | 0 | 1 | 2 | 0 |
| | | | | | | |
| 15 | 61 | 1 | 0.5 | 1 | 1 | 0 |

| MILK AND MILK SUBSTITUTES | AVERAGE PORTION g |
|---|---|
| Skimmed milk, pasteurised | 146 |
| Skimmed milk, sterilised | 136 |
| Skimmed milk, UHT | 146 |
| Soya milk | 146 |
| Soya milk, flavoured | 146 |
| Whole milk, dried | 3 |
| Whole milk, pasteurised | 146 |
| Whole milk, sterilised | 146 |
| Whole milk, UHT | 146 |

## YOGHURTS

| | |
|---|---|
| Crème fraîche (see under cream) | |
| Fromage frais (see under cheese) | |
| Drinking yoghurt | 200 |
| Probiotic yoghurt drink, orange | 100 |
| Probiotic yoghurt drink, plain | 100 |
| Yoghurt, French set, fruit, low-fat | 125 |
| Yoghurt, fruit | 125 |
| Yoghurt, fruit, low-fat | 125 |
| Yoghurt, fruit, virtuallly fat-free | 125 |
| Yoghurt, Greek-style, fruit, whole milk | 150 |
| Yoghurt, Greek-style, honey, whole milk | 150 |
| Yoghurt, Greek-style, natural, whole milk | 150 |
| Yoghurt, hazelnut, low-fat | 125 |
| Yoghurt, long life, fruit, whole milk | 125 |
| Yoghurt, natural, low-fat | 125 |
| Yoghurt, natural, virtually fat-free | 125 |
| Yoghurt, soya, fruit | 125 |
| Yoghurt, toffee, low-fat | 125 |
| Yoghurt, twin pot, fruit, virtually fat-free | 135 |
| Yoghurt, vanilla, low-fat | 125 |

Unless otherwise specified, milk is cows' milk.

| ENERGY kcal | ENERGY kJ | FAT g | SATURATED FAT g | PROTEIN g | CARBOHYDRATE g | FIBRE g |
|---|---|---|---|---|---|---|
| 48 | 204 | 1 | 0.1 | 5 | 7 | 0 |
| 44 | 188 | 1 | 0.1 | 5 | 7 | 0 |
| 47 | 200 | 1 | 0.1 | 5 | 7 | 0 |
| 47 | 193 | 2 | 0.4 | 4 | 1 | Trace |
| 58 | 245 | 2 | 0.3 | 4 | 5 | Trace |
| 15 | 62 | 1 | 0.5 | 1 | 1 | 0 |
| 96 | 402 | 6 | 3.5 | 5 | 7 | 0 |
| 96 | 404 | 6 | 3.5 | 5 | 7 | 0 |
| 96 | 402 | 6 | 3.5 | 5 | 7 | 0 |
| 124 | 526 | Trace | Trace | 6 | 26 | Trace |
| 67 | 279 | 0.9 | 0.6 | 1.5 | 13.4 | 1.3 |
| 68 | 284 | 1 | 0.7 | 1.7 | 13.1 | 1.4 |
| 103 | 435 | 1.4 | 1.0 | 4.3 | 19.5 | 0.3 |
| 133 | 564 | 3.8 | 2.5 | 4.9 | 21.4 | 0.3 |
| 97 | 412 | 1.4 | 0.9 | 5.1 | 17.1 | 0.3 |
| 75 | 318 | 0.5 | 0.0 | 5.9 | 12.5 | 0.3 |
| 205 | 857 | 12.6 | 8.4 | 7.2 | 16.8 | Trace |
| 221 | 927 | 12.5 | 8.4 | 7.7 | 21.0 | Trace |
| 198 | 824 | 15.3 | 10.2 | 8.4 | 7.2 | Trace |
| 111 | 469 | 1.9 | 0.8 | 5.5 | 19.1 | 0.3 |
| 125 | 529 | 4.3 | 0.0 | 3.9 | 19.1 | 0.3 |
| 69 | 294 | 1.3 | 0.9 | 5.9 | 9.3 | Trace |
| 67 | 286 | 0.3 | 0.0 | 6.6 | 10.3 | Trace |
| 92 | 388 | 2.3 | 0.3 | 2.9 | 16.0 | 0.4 |
| 114 | 484 | 1.1 | 0.8 | 4.8 | 22.6 | Trace |
| 55 | 236 | 0.1 | 0.1 | 4.5 | 9.7 | 0.7 |
| 114 | 484 | 1.1 | 0.8 | 4.8 | 22.6 | Trace |

DAIRY
PRODUCTS 93

| FATS | AVERAGE PORTION g |
|---|---|
| **Butter** | |
| Butter | 20 |
| Ghee | 7 |
| **Margarine** | |
| Hard, animal and vegetable fats | 10 |
| Hard, vegetable fats | 10 |
| Soft, animal and vegetable fat | 7 |
| Soft, polyunsaturated | 7 |
| **Other fats** | |
| Compound cooking fat | 15 |
| Compound cooking fat, polyunsaturated | 15 |
| Dripping, beef | 15 |
| Ghee, vegetable | 7 |
| Lard | 15 |
| Suet, beef, shredded | 15 |
| Suet, vegetable | 15 |
| **Spreads** | |
| Blended 70% fat | 7 |
| Blended 40% fat | 7 |
| 20–25% fat, not polyunsaturated | 7 |
| 20–25% fat | 7 |
| 35–40% fat | 7 |
| 40% fat, not polyunsaturated | 7 |
| 5% fat | 7 |
| 60% fat | 7 |
| 60% fat, with olive oil | 7 |
| 70% fat | 7 |

| OILS | |
|---|---|
| Corn oil | 15 |
| Grapeseed oil | 11 |
| Hazelnut oil | 2 |

| ENERGY kcal | ENERGY kJ | FAT g | SATURATED FAT g | PROTEIN g | CARBOHYDRATE g | FIBRE g |
|---|---|---|---|---|---|---|
| 147 | 606 | 16 | 11 | 0 | Trace | 0 |
| 63 | 259 | 7 | 4.6 | Trace | Trace | 0 |
| | | | | | | |
| 72 | 295 | 8 | 3.5 | 0 | 0 | 0 |
| 74 | 304 | 8 | 3.6 | 0 | 0 | 0 |
| 52 | 213 | 6 | 1.9 | 0 | 0 | 0 |
| 52 | 215 | 6 | 1.2 | Trace | 0 | 0 |
| | | | | | | |
| 135 | 554 | 15 | 7.4 | Trace | 0 | 0 |
| | | | | | | |
| 135 | 554 | 15 | 3.1 | Trace | Trace | 0 |
| 134 | 549 | 15 | 7.9 | Trace | Trace | 0 |
| 63 | 257 | 7 | 3.4 | Trace | Trace | 0 |
| 134 | 549 | 15 | 6 | Trace | 0 | 0 |
| 124 | 510 | 14 | 7.5 | Trace | 2 | 0.1 |
| 125 | 517 | 13 | 6.8 | 0 | 2 | 0 |
| | | | | | | |
| 48 | 196 | 5 | 1.8 | 0 | 0 | 0 |
| 27 | 113 | 3 | 1.3 | 0 | 0 | 0 |
| 17 | 71 | 2 | 0.4 | 0 | 0 | 0 |
| 13 | 53 | 1 | 0.3 | 0 | 0 | 0 |
| 26 | 105 | 3 | 0.6 | 0 | 0 | 0 |
| 28 | 113 | 3 | 0.8 | 0 | 0 | 0 |
| 7 | 30 | 1 | 0.1 | 0 | 1 | 0.4 |
| 39 | 159 | 4 | 0.8 | 0 | 0 | 0 |
| 40 | 164 | 4 | 0.8 | 0 | 0 | 0 |
| 44 | 183 | 5 | 0.9 | 0 | 0 | 0 |
| | | | | | | |
| 135 | 554 | 15 | 2.2 | Trace | 0 | 0 |
| 99 | 407 | 11 | 1.2 | Trace | 0 | 0 |
| 99 | 407 | 11 | 0.9 | Trace | 0 | 0 |

| **OILS** | AVERAGE PORTION g |
|---|---|
| Olive oil | 11 |
| Palm oil | 11 |
| Peanut oil | 11 |
| Rapeseed oil | 11 |
| Safflower oil | 11 |
| Sesame oil | 3 |
| Soya oil | 11 |
| Sunflower oil | 11 |
| Vegetable oil | 11 |
| Walnut oil | 11 |
| Wheatgerm oil | 11 |

| ENERGY kcal | ENERGY kJ | FAT g | SATURATED FAT g | PROTEIN g | CARBOHYDRATE g | FIBRE g |
|---|---|---|---|---|---|---|
| 99 | 407 | 11 | 1.6 | Trace | 0 | 0 |
| 99 | 407 | 11 | 5.3 | Trace | 0 | 0 |
| 99 | 407 | 11 | 2.2 | Trace | 0 | 0 |
| 99 | 407 | 11 | 0.7 | Trace | 0 | 0 |
| 99 | 407 | 11 | 1.1 | Trace | 0 | 0 |
| 27 | 111 | 3 | 0.4 | Trace | 0 | 0 |
| 99 | 407 | 11 | 1.7 | Trace | 0 | 0 |
| 99 | 407 | 11 | 1.3 | Trace | 0 | 0 |
| 99 | 407 | 11 | 1.1 | Trace | 0 | 0 |
| 99 | 407 | 11 | 1 | Trace | 0 | 0 |
| 99 | 407 | 11 | 2 | Trace | 0 | 0 |

| SWEET SPREADS | AVERAGE PORTION g |
|---|---|
| Chocolate spread | 16 |
| Fruit spread | 16 |
| Honey | 17 |
| Lemon curd | 15 |

## SAVOURY SPREADS AND PATES

| | |
|---|---|
| Fish paste | 10 |
| Mackerel pâté, smoked | 40 |
| Meat extract | 9 |
| Meat spread | 10 |
| Liver sausage | 40 |
| Pâté, liver, tubed | 40 |
| Peanut butter, smooth | 25 |
| Peanut butter, crunchy | 25 |
| Sandwich spread | 15 |
| Tofu spread | 45 |
| Tuna pâté | 40 |
| Vegetable pâté | 80 |
| Yeast extract | 9 |

## JAMS AND MARMALADES

| | |
|---|---|
| Jam, diabetic | 15 |
| Jam, fruit with edible seeds | 15 |
| Jam, reduced sugar | 15 |
| Jam, stone fruit | 15 |
| Marmalade | 15 |
| Marmalade, diabetic | 15 |

Unless otherwise specified, spreads are made with polyunsaturated fats.

| ENERGY kcal | ENERGY kJ | FAT g | SATURATED FAT g | PROTEIN g | CARBOHYDRATE g | FIBRE g |
|---|---|---|---|---|---|---|
| 91 | 380 | 6 | 0.9 | 1 | 9 | 0.2 |
| 19 | 83 | Trace | Trace | 0 | 5 | 0.1 |
| 49 | 209 | 0 | 0 | 0 | 13 | 0 |
| 42 | 180 | 1 | 0.2 | 0 | 9 | 0 |
| | | | | | | |
| 17 | 71 | 1 | 0.5 | 2 | 0 | 0 |
| 147 | 608 | 14 | 2.5 | 5 | 1 | Trace |
| 16 | 68 | 0 | 0 | 4 | 0 | 0 |
| 19 | 80 | 1 | 0.6 | 2 | 0 | Trace |
| 90 | 377 | 7 | 2.1 | 5 | 2 | 0.3 |
| 114 | 472 | 10 | 3 | 5 | 0 | Trace |
| 156 | 645 | 13 | 2.9 | 6 | 3 | 1.4 |
| 152 | 628 | 13 | 2.4 | 6 | 2 | 1.5 |
| 28 | 117 | 1 | 0.2 | 0 | 4 | 0.1 |
| 94 | 349 | 9 | 1.3 | 2 | 1 | 0.2 |
| 94 | 393 | 7 | 3.1 | 7 | 0 | Trace |
| 138 | 574 | 11 | 6 | 6 | 5 | 2 |
| 16 | 69 | 0 | 0 | 4 | 0 | 0 |
| | | | | | | |
| 26 | 109 | 0 | 0 | 0 | 9 | 0.1 |
| 39 | 167 | 0 | 0 | 0 | 10 | 0.1 |
| 18 | 78 | Trace | Trace | 0 | 5 | 0.1 |
| 39 | 167 | 0 | 0 | 0 | 10 | 0.1 |
| 39 | 167 | 0 | 0 | 0 | 10 | 0 |
| 26 | 109 | 0 | 0 | 0 | 9 | 0.1 |

| BREAKFAST CEREALS | AVERAGE PORTION g |
|---|---|
| Bran, flakes | 30 |
| Bran, flakes with oat | 30 |
| Bran, strands | 40 |
| Bran, sultana | 30 |
| Bran, with oat and wheat | 50 |
| Corn flakes | 30 |
| Corn flakes, with nuts | 30 |
| Crunchy clusters with fruit | 50 |
| Crunchy clusters with chocolate | 50 |
| Frosted flakes | 30 |
| Fruit and fibre breakfast cereal | 40 |
| Hoops, honey | 30 |
| Hoops, honey and nut | 30 |
| Malted flakes | 30 |
| Muesli | 50 |
| Muesli, Swiss-style | 50 |
| Muesli, with extra fruit | 50 |
| Muesli, with no added sugar | 50 |
| Multigrain flakes | 30 |
| Oat cereal with fruit and nuts | 50 |
| Oat cereal with tropical fruit | 50 |
| Oat clusters | 30 |
| Oat flakes | 30 |
| Porridge, instant, made with water | 180 |
| Porridge, made with milk and water | 160 |
| Porridge, made with water | 160 |
| Porridge, made with whole milk | 160 |
| Puffed wheat | 20 |
| Rice pops | 30 |
| Rice pops, chocolate | 30 |
| Wheat, shredded | 45 |
| Wheat, shredded, honey and nut | 40 |
| Wheat, shredded, mini | 45 |
| Wholewheat biscuits | 20 |

All values are without any sugar added.

| ENERGY kcal | ENERGY kJ | FAT g | SATURATED FAT g | PROTEIN g | CARBOHYDRATE g | FIBRE g |
|---|---|---|---|---|---|---|
| 95 | 406 | 1 | 0.1 | 3 | 21 | 3.9 |
| 105 | 435 | 2 | 0.2 | 3 | 20 | 3 |
| 104 | 444 | 1 | 0.2 | 6 | 19 | 9.8 |
| 96 | 405 | 1 | 0.1 | 3 | 18 | 3.9 |
| 163 | 691 | 2 | 0.3 | 5 | 34 | 8.9 |
| 108 | 461 | Trace | 0 | 2 | 26 | 0.3 |
| 119 | 507 | 1 | 0.2 | 2 | 27 | 0.2 |
| 139 | 580 | 5 | 1.7 | 4 | 20 | 1.3 |
| 220 | 917 | 8 | 2.7 | 3 | 33 | 2.4 |
| 113 | 482 | Trace | 0 | 2 | 28 | 0.2 |
| 147 | 614 | 2 | 1.2 | 2 | 28 | 2.2 |
| 111 | 465 | 1 | 0.2 | 2 | 23 | 2.1 |
| 112 | 474 | 1 | 0.3 | 2 | 23 | 1.5 |
| 186 | 773 | 1 | 0.1 | 3 | 23 | 1.3 |
| 184 | 770 | 3 | 0.7 | 6 | 33 | 3.2 |
| 182 | 770 | 3 | 0.4 | 5 | 36 | 3.2 |
| 186 | 789 | 3 | 0.4 | 5 | 37 | 3.2 |
| 183 | 776 | 4 | 0.8 | 5 | 34 | 3.8 |
| 111 | 465 | Trace | Trace | 5 | 22 | 0.7 |
| 213 | 888 | 8 | 3 | 5 | 31 | 2 |
| 217 | 905 | 7 | 4 | 4 | 34 | 3 |
| 116 | 490 | 3 | 0.8 | 3 | 20 | 2.7 |
| 107 | 456 | 1 | 0.2 | 3 | 22 | 3 |
| 671 | 2844 | 14 | 2.2 | 21 | 123 | 13 |
| 133 | 557 | 5 | 2.3 | 5 | 18 | 1.3 |
| 78 | 334 | 2 | 0.3 | 2 | 14 | 1.3 |
| 186 | 781 | 8 | 4.3 | 8 | 22 | 1.3 |
| 64 | 273 | Trace | 0 | 3 | 13 | 1.1 |
| 111 | 472 | 0.1 | 0.1 | 2 | 27 | 0.2 |
| 115 | 491 | 0.1 | 0.1 | 2 | 28 | 0.2 |
| 150 | 630 | 1 | 0.2 | 5 | 30 | 5.2 |
| 152 | 642 | 3 | 0.9 | 4 | 28 | 4.1 |
| 154 | 655 | 1 | 0.2 | 4 | 32 | 5 |
| 70 | 300 | 0.1 | 0.1 | 2 | 15 | 1.9 |

| SAVOURY BISCUITS | AVERAGE PORTION g |
|---|---|
| Cheese sandwiches | 24 |
| Cream crackers | 14 |
| Oatcakes, shop bought | 26 |
| Water biscuits | 16 |
| Wholemeal crackers | 20 |

| CRISPBREADS | |
|---|---|
| Breadsticks (4) | 28 |
| Crispbakes | 16 |
| Crispbread, rye | 20 |
| French toast | 16 |
| Matzos | 20 |
| Melba toast | 6 |
| Rice cakes | 16 |

| SWEET BISCUITS | |
|---|---|
| All-butter biscuits | 19 |
| Bourbon creams | 28 |
| Brandy snaps | 30 |
| Chocolate, full-coated | 50 |
| Chocolate-covered teacakes | 26 |
| Coconut biscuits | 40 |
| Cookies, chocolate chip | 22 |
| Cookies, chocolate chip and hazelnut (1) | 24 |
| Cookies, Danish butter | 22 |
| Cookies, stem ginger | 32 |
| Crunch biscuits | 27 |
| Custard creams | 24 |
| Custard creams, reduced fat | 24 |
| Digestives, chocolate, half coated | 26 |
| Digestives, milk chocolate, reduced fat | 34 |

Unless otherwise specified, a helping is two biscuits.

| ENERGY kcal | ENERGY kJ | FAT g | SATURATED FAT g | PROTEIN g | CARBOHYDRATE g | FIBRE g |
|---|---|---|---|---|---|---|
| 123 | 516 | 5 | 3.5 | 1 | 17 | 0.2 |
| 62 | 260 | 2 | 0.4 | 1 | 10 | 0.3 |
| 115 | 482 | 4 | 1 | 3 | 16 | 1.3 |
| 70 | 297 | 1 | Trace | 2 | 12 | 0.5 |
| 83 | 349 | 2 | 1 | 2 | 14 | 0.9 |
| | | | | | | |
| 108 | 464 | 4 | 1.6 | 4 | 20 | 0.8 |
| 60 | 250 | Trace | Trace | 2 | 12 | 0.6 |
| 64 | 273 | 0.1 | 0.1 | 2 | 14 | 2.3 |
| 63 | 262 | 1 | 0.5 | 2 | 12 | 0.5 |
| 77 | 327 | 0 | 0 | 2 | 17 | 0.6 |
| 23 | 94 | Trace | Trace | 1 | 4 | 0.3 |
| 56 | 234 | Trace | Trace | 2 | 12 | 0.8 |
| | | | | | | |
| 90 | 378 | 4 | 3.4 | Trace | 14 | 0.2 |
| 136 | 566 | 6 | 3.6 | 2 | 20 | 0.6 |
| 131 | 550 | 6 | 3 | 1 | 19 | 0.2 |
| 262 | 1099 | 13 | 8.4 | 3 | 34 | 1 |
| 116 | 438 | 4 | 2.2 | 2 | 16 | 0.4 |
| 202 | 846 | 12 | 6 | 2 | 21 | 2 |
| 112 | 461 | 6 | 2.7 | 1 | 14 | 0.4 |
| 120 | 504 | 6 | 2.6 | 2 | 14 | 0.4 |
| 112 | 461 | 5 | 4 | 1 | 14 | 0.3 |
| 157 | 653 | 9 | 1.9 | 1 | 20 | 0.6 |
| 135 | 562 | 7 | 3.5 | 2 | 17 | 0.6 |
| 122 | 508 | 6 | 3.6 | 2 | 16 | 0.4 |
| 114 | 472 | 4 | 2.6 | 2 | 18 | 0.4 |
| | | | | | | |
| 128 | 538 | 6 | 3.2 | 2 | 17 | 0.6 |
| 158 | 660 | 10 | 6 | 2 | 24 | 0.6 |

| SWEET BISCUITS | AVERAGE PORTION g |
|---|---|
| Digestives, plain | 26 |
| Digestives, reduced fat | 28 |
| Flapjacks (1 piece) | 70 |
| Gingernuts | 20 |
| Jaffa cakes | 26 |
| Jam rings | 38 |
| Jam sandwich creams | 30 |
| Malted milk | 16 |
| Malted milk creams | 26 |
| Marshmallow teacakes, chocolate-coated | 28 |
| Morning coffee | 10 |
| Nice | 20 |
| Nice creams | 28 |
| Rich tea | 14 |
| Shortbread | 26 |
| Shortbread, chocolate chip | 40 |
| Shortbread, reduced sugar (1) | 33 |
| Snowballs | 42 |
| Wafers, filled | 14 |

Unless otherwise specified, a helping is two biscuits.

| ENERGY kcal | ENERGY kJ | FAT g | SATURATED FAT g | PROTEIN g | CARBOHYDRATE g | FIBRE g |
|---|---|---|---|---|---|---|
| 122 | 514 | 5 | 2.2 | 2 | 18 | 0.6 |
| 130 | 542 | 6 | 2 | 2 | 20 | 1 |
| 339 | 1420 | 19 | 5.3 | 3 | 42 | 1.9 |
| 91 | 385 | 3 | 1.4 | 1 | 16 | 0.3 |
| 94 | 398 | 3 | 0.6 | 1 | 18 | 0.4 |
| 171 | 715 | 6 | 2.7 | 2 | 27 | 0.6 |
| 142 | 592 | 6 | 3.2 | 2 | 20 | 0.6 |
| 78 | 324 | 3 | 1.8 | 1 | 11 | 0.3 |
| 130 | 542 | 6 | 3.7 | 2 | 17 | 0.4 |
| | | | | | | |
| 126 | 525 | 5 | 3 | 1 | 18 | 0.4 |
| 45 | 188 | 1 | 0.6 | 1 | 7 | 0.2 |
| 94 | 393 | 4 | 2.3 | 1 | 12 | 0.3 |
| 140 | 584 | 6 | 3.2 | 2 | 18 | 0.6 |
| 64 | 270 | 2 | 1.1 | 1 | 10 | 0.2 |
| 129 | 543 | 7 | 4.5 | 2 | 17 | 0.5 |
| 206 | 858 | 10 | 8.6 | 2 | 24 | 0.6 |
| 156 | 652 | 9 | 5.9 | 2 | 18 | 0.5 |
| 196 | 814 | 10 | 9.8 | 2 | 24 | 2.2 |
| 75 | 314 | 4 | 2.6 | 1 | 9 | 0.3 |

| SAVOURY SNACKS | AVERAGE PORTION g |
|---|---|
| Bacon streaks | 25 |
| Bombay mix | 30 |
| Breadsticks | 28 |
| Cheese and potato puffs | 27 |
| Cheese balls | 33 |
| Corn snacks | 28 |
| Oriental mix | 50 |
| Popcorn, candied | 75 |
| Popcorn, salted | 75 |
| Pork scratchings | 22 |
| Potato and corn sticks | 19 |
| Potato and corn, waffle-shaped snacks | 50 |
| Potato crisps | 30 |
| Potato crisps, crinkle cut | 40 |
| Potato crisps, jacket | 40 |
| Potato crisps, low-fat | 30 |
| Potato crisps, square | 25 |
| Potato crisps, thick, crinkle cut | 40 |
| Potato crisps, thick cut | 40 |
| Potato rings | 30 |
| Prawn crackers | 20 |
| Pretzels | 30 |
| Punjabi puri | 35 |
| Tortilla chips | 50 |
| Trail mix | 25 |
| Twiglets | 25 |
| Wheat crunchies | 35 |

| ENERGY kcal | ENERGY kJ | FAT g | SATURATED FAT g | PROTEIN g | CARBOHYDRATE g | FIBRE g |
|---|---|---|---|---|---|---|
| 113 | 473 | 5 | 1.6 | 2 | 16 | 0.5 |
| 151 | 630 | 10 | 1.2 | 6 | 11 | 1.9 |
| 108 | 464 | 4 | 1.6 | 4 | 20 | 0.8 |
| 140 | 585 | 9 | 3.2 | 2 | 15 | 0.3 |
| 148 | 621 | 8 | 1.8 | 2 | 19 | 0.8 |
| 141 | 591 | 9 | 3.8 | 1 | 16 | 1 |
| 273 | 1142 | 20 | 3 | 10 | 17 | 0.3 |
| 360 | 1514 | 14 | 1.5 | 2 | 58 | 1 |
| 445 | 1851 | 32 | 3.2 | 5 | 37 | 1 |
| 133 | 554 | 10 | 3.6 | 11 | 0 | 0.1 |
| 88 | 368 | 4 | 1.3 | 1 | 11 | 0.6 |
| 241 | 1009 | 12 | 2.8 | 2 | 32 | 1.3 |
| 159 | 665 | 10 | 4.2 | 2 | 16 | 1.6 |
| 219 | 913 | 14 | 5.8 | 2 | 22 | 2.3 |
| 204 | 851 | 13 | 5.3 | 3 | 21 | 1.9 |
| 137 | 577 | 6 | 2.8 | 2 | 19 | 1.8 |
| 108 | 454 | 5 | 2.2 | 2 | 14 | 1.1 |
| 203 | 848 | 12 | 5 | 2 | 22 | 1.6 |
| 200 | 836 | 11 | 4.6 | 3 | 23 | 1.6 |
| 157 | 656 | 10 | 4.2 | 1 | 18 | 0.8 |
| 103 | 432 | 7 | 1.9 | 0 | 11 | 0.3 |
| 114 | 479 | 1 | 0.2 | 3 | 24 | 0.8 |
| 188 | 784 | 12 | 2.9 | 3 | 18 | 0.9 |
| 230 | 964 | 11 | 2 | 4 | 30 | 3 |
| 108 | 451 | 7 | 1.3 | 2 | 9 | 1.1 |
| 96 | 404 | 3 | 1.2 | 3 | 16 | 2.6 |
| 158 | 662 | 7 | 3.2 | 4 | 21 | 1.2 |

| | AVERAGE PORTION g |
|---|---|
| **FLOUR** | |
| Chapati, brown | 100 |
| Chapati, white | 100 |
| Cornflour | 30 |
| Rye, whole | 20 |
| Wheat, brown | 100 |
| Wheat, white, breadmaking | 100 |
| Wheat, white, plain | 100 |
| Wheat, white, self-raising | 100 |
| Wheat, wholemeal | 100 |
| | |
| **GRAVY AND STOCK CUBES** | |
| Instant granules | 5 |
| Instant granules, made up | 45 |
| Stock cubes, beef/chicken | 7 |
| Stock cubes, vegetable | 7 |
| | |
| **BAKING INGREDIENTS** | |
| Baking powder | 4 |
| Marzipan, shop bought | 25 |
| Mincemeat | 28 |
| Mincemeat, vegetarian | 28 |
| Yeast, bakers', compressed | 5 |
| Yeast, dried | 5 |
| | |
| **MISCELLANEOUS** | |
| Bran, wheat | 7 |
| Coconut, creamed block | 25 |
| Coconut, desiccated | 28 |
| Custard powder | 30 |
| Gelatine | 3 |
| Olives, in brine, stoned | 18 |

| ENERGY kcal | ENERGY kJ | FAT g | SATURATED FAT g | PROTEIN g | CARBOHYDRATE g | FIBRE g |
|---|---|---|---|---|---|---|
| 333 | 1419 | 1 | 0.2 | 12 | 74 | 6 |
| 335 | 1426 | 1 | 0.1 | 10 | 78 | 3 |
| 106 | 452 | 0 | 0 | 0 | 28 | 0 |
| 67 | 286 | 1 | 0.1 | 2 | 15 | 2.3 |
| 323 | 1377 | 2 | 0.2 | 13 | 69 | 6.4 |
| 341 | 1451 | 1 | 0.2 | 12 | 75 | 3.1 |
| 341 | 1450 | 1 | 0.2 | 9 | 78 | 3.1 |
| 330 | 1407 | 1 | 0.2 | 9 | 76 | 3.1 |
| 310 | 1318 | 2 | 0.3 | 13 | 64 | 9 |
| | | | | | | |
| 23 | 96 | 2 | Trace | 0 | 2 | Trace |
| 15 | 64 | 1 | Trace | 0 | 1 | Trace |
| 17 | 69 | 1 | Trace | 1 | 1 | 0 |
| 18 | 74 | 1 | Trace | 1 | 1 | Trace |
| | | | | | | |
| 7 | 28 | 0 | 0 | 0 | 2 | 0 |
| 101 | 426 | 3 | 0.3 | 1 | 17 | 0.5 |
| 77 | 326 | 1 | Trace | 0 | 17 | 0.4 |
| 85 | 359 | 4 | Trace | 0 | 12 | 0.4 |
| 3 | 11 | 0 | 0 | 1 | 0 | Trace |
| 8 | 36 | 0 | 0 | 2 | 0 | Trace |
| | | | | | | |
| 14 | 61 | 1 | 0.1 | 1 | 2 | 2.5 |
| 167 | 690 | 17 | 14.8 | 2 | 2 | 2 |
| 169 | 698 | 17 | 15 | 2 | 2 | 3.8 |
| 106 | 452 | 0 | 0 | 0 | 28 | 0 |
| 10 | 43 | 0 | 0 | 3 | 0 | 0 |
| 19 | 76 | 2 | 0.3 | 0 | Trace | 0.5 |

STORECUPBOARD
INGREDIENTS

## MISCELLANEOUS

| | AVERAGE PORTION g |
|---|---|
| Salt | 5 |
| Tomatoes, sundried, bottled in oil | 10 |
| Vinegar | 15 |
| Wheatgerm | 5 |

## PURÉES

| | |
|---|---|
| Tomato purée | 20 |
| Vegetable purée | 20 |

## SUGARS, SYRUPS AND TREACLE

| | |
|---|---|
| Jaggery | 16 |
| Sugar, brown | 20 |
| Sugar, Demerara | 20 |
| Sugar, icing | 20 |
| Sugar, white | 20 |
| Syrup, golden | 55 |
| Syrup, golden, pouring | 50 |
| Syrup, maple | 55 |
| Treacle, black | 50 |

## NUTS AND SEEDS

| | |
|---|---|
| Almonds, toasted | 13 |
| Barcelona nuts | 15 |
| Brazil nuts | 10 |
| Cashew nuts, plain | 10 |
| Cashew nuts, roasted and salted | 25 |
| Chestnuts | 50 |
| Coconut, fresh | 28 |
| Hazelnuts | 10 |
| Macadamia nuts, salted | 10 |
| Melon seeds | 15 |

| ENERGY kcal | ENERGY kJ | FAT g | SATURATED FAT g | PROTEIN g | CARBOHYDRATE g | FIBRE g |
|---|---|---|---|---|---|---|
| 0 | 0 | 0 | 0 | 0 | 0 | 0 |
| 50 | 204 | 5 | 0.7 | 0 | 1 | 0.5 |
| 3 | 13 | 0 | 0 | 0 | 0 | 0 |
| 18 | 75 | 0 | 0.1 | 1 | 2 | 0.8 |
| | | | | | | |
| 15 | 65 | Trace | Trace | 1 | 3 | 0.6 |
| 14 | 51 | 1 | 0 | 1 | 1 | 0.6 |
| | | | | | | |
| 59 | 250 | 0 | 0 | 0 | 16 | 0 |
| 72 | 309 | 0 | 0 | 0 | 20 | 0 |
| 79 | 336 | 0 | 0 | 0 | 21 | 0 |
| 79 | 336 | 0 | 0 | Trace | 21 | 0 |
| 79 | 336 | 0 | 0 | Trace | 21 | 0 |
| 164 | 698 | 0 | 0 | 0 | 43 | 0 |
| 148 | 632 | 0 | 0 | Trace | 40 | 0 |
| 144 | 602 | Trace | Trace | 0 | 37 | 0 |
| 129 | 548 | 0 | 0 | 1 | 34 | Trace |
| | | | | | | |
| 81 | 334 | 7 | 0.6 | 3 | 1 | 1 |
| 96 | 396 | 10 | 2.3 | 2 | 1 | 1 |
| 68 | 281 | 7 | 1.6 | 1 | 0 | 0.4 |
| 57 | 237 | 5 | 1 | 2 | 2 | 0.3 |
| 153 | 633 | 13 | 2.5 | 5 | 5 | 0.8 |
| 85 | 360 | 1 | 0.3 | 1 | 18 | 2 |
| 98 | 405 | 10 | 8.7 | 1 | 1 | 2 |
| 65 | 269 | 6 | 0.5 | 1 | 1 | 0.7 |
| 75 | 308 | 8 | 1.1 | 1 | 0 | 0.5 |
| 87 | 363 | 7 | 1.8 | 4 | 1 | 0.8 |

STORECUPBOARD
INGREDIENTS 11

| NUTS AND SEEDS | AVERAGE PORTION g |
| --- | --- |
| Mixed nuts | 40 |
| Mixed nuts and raisins | 40 |
| Peanuts, dry roasted | 40 |
| Peanuts, plain | 13 |
| Peanuts, roasted and salted | 25 |
| Pecan nuts | 60 |
| Pine nuts | 5 |
| Pistachio nuts, roasted and salted | 10 |
| Pumpkin seeds | 16 |
| Sesame seeds | 12 |
| Sunflower seeds | 16 |
| Walnuts | 20 |

| ENERGY kcal | ENERGY kJ | FAT g | SATURATED FAT g | PROTEIN g | CARBOHYDRATE g | FIBRE g |
|---|---|---|---|---|---|---|
| 243 | 1006 | 22 | 3.4 | 9 | 3 | 2.4 |
| 192 | 802 | 14 | 2.2 | 6 | 13 | 1.8 |
| 236 | 976 | 20 | 3.6 | 10 | 4 | 2.6 |
| 73 | 304 | 6 | 1.1 | 3 | 2 | 0.8 |
| 151 | 623 | 13 | 2.4 | 6 | 2 | 1.5 |
| 413 | 1706 | 42 | 3.4 | 6 | 3 | 2.8 |
| 34 | 142 | 3 | 0.2 | 1 | 0 | 0.1 |
| 60 | 249 | 6 | 0.7 | 2 | 1 | 0.6 |
| 91 | 378 | 7 | 1.1 | 4 | 2 | 0.8 |
| 72 | 296 | 7 | 1 | 2 | 0 | 0.9 |
| 96 | 400 | 8 | 0.8 | 3 | 3 | 1 |
| 138 | 567 | 14 | 1.1 | 3 | 1 | 0.7 |

| TABLE SAUCES | AVERAGE PORTION g |
|---|---|
| Apple sauce, homemade | 20 |
| Brown sauce | 20 |
| Brown sauce, hot | 20 |
| Brown sauce, sweet | 20 |
| Chilli sauce | 25 |
| Horseradish sauce | 20 |
| Mint sauce | 10 |
| Mustard, powder, made up | 8 |
| Mustard, smooth | 2 |
| Mustard, wholegrain | 14 |
| Soy sauce, dark, thick | 5 |
| Soy sauce, light, thin | 5 |
| Tartare sauce | 30 |
| Tomato ketchup | 20 |

| WHITE SAUCES | |
|---|---|
| Bread sauce, made with semi-skimmed milk | 45 |
| Bread sauce, made with whole milk | 45 |
| Cheese sauce, made with semi-skimmed milk | 62 |
| Cheese sauce, made with whole milk | 62 |
| Onion sauce, made with semi-skimmed milk | 62 |
| Onion sauce, made with whole milk | 62 |
| White sauce, savoury, made with semi-skimmed milk | 62 |
| White sauce, savoury, made with whole milk | 62 |
| White sauce, sweet, made with semi-skimmed milk | 62 |
| White sauce, sweet, made with whole milk | 62 |

| ENERGY kcal | ENERGY kJ | FAT g | SATURATED FAT g | PROTEIN g | CARBOHYDRATE g | FIBRE g |
|---|---|---|---|---|---|---|
| 13 | 55 | 0 | 0 | 0 | 3 | 0.2 |
| 20 | 84 | Trace | Trace | 0 | 5 | 0.1 |
| 24 | 102 | Trace | Trace | 0 | 6 | 0.1 |
| 20 | 84 | Trace | Trace | 0 | 4 | 0.1 |
| 20 | 84 | Trace | Trace | 0 | 4 | 0.3 |
| 31 | 128 | 2 | 0.2 | 1 | 4 | 0.5 |
| 10 | 43 | Trace | Trace | 0 | 2 | 0.2 |
| 18 | 75 | 1 | 0.1 | 1 | 0 | 0 |
| 3 | 12 | 0 | 0 | 0 | 0 | 0 |
| 20 | 82 | 1 | 0.1 | 1 | 5 | Trace |
| 3 | 13 | 0 | 0 | 0 | 6 | 0.2 |
| 3 | 13 | Trace | Trace | 0 | 1 | 0.7 |
| 90 | 372 | 7 | 0.5 | 0 | 0 | 0.2 |
| 23 | 98 | Trace | Trace | 0 | 1 | 0.7 |
| | | | | | | |
| 42 | 177 | 1 | 0.6 | 2 | 6 | 0.1 |
| 50 | 208 | 2 | 1.2 | 2 | 6 | 0.1 |
| | | | | | | |
| 112 | 465 | 8 | 3.9 | 4 | 6 | 0.1 |
| 122 | 508 | 8 | 4.8 | 4 | 6 | 0.1 |
| | | | | | | |
| 53 | 224 | 3 | 1.1 | 2 | 5 | 0.2 |
| 61 | 257 | 4 | 1.7 | 2 | 5 | 0.2 |
| | | | | | | |
| 79 | 334 | 5 | 1.8 | 3 | 7 | 0.1 |
| | | | | | | |
| 93 | 387 | 6 | 2.7 | 3 | 7 | 0.1 |
| | | | | | | |
| 93 | 393 | 4 | 1.7 | 2 | 12 | 0.1 |
| | | | | | | |
| 105 | 441 | 6 | 2.5 | 2 | 12 | 0.1 |

## CHUTNEYS

|  | AVERAGE PORTION g |
|---|---|
| Chutney, apple, homemade | 33 |
| Chutney, mango, oily | 33 |
| Chutney, mango, sweet | 33 |
| Chutney, mixed fruit | 33 |
| Chutney, tomato | 33 |

## DIPS

| | |
|---|---|
| Dips, sour-cream-based | 30 |
| Guacamole | 45 |
| Hummus | 30 |
| Taramasalata | 45 |
| Tzatziki | 45 |

## DRESSINGS

| | |
|---|---|
| Blue cheese | 25 |
| 'Fat-free' | 15 |
| French | 15 |
| Low-fat | 15 |
| Oil and lemon | 15 |
| Thousand island | 30 |
| Thousand island, reduced-calorie | 30 |
| Yogurt-based | 30 |

## MAYONNAISE AND SALAD CREAM

| | |
|---|---|
| Mayonnaise | 30 |
| Mayonnaise, homemade, made with lemon juice | 30 |
| Mayonnaise, homemade, made with vinegar | 30 |
| Mayonnaise, reduced-calorie | 30 |

| ENERGY kcal | ENERGY kJ | FAT g | SATURATED FAT g | PROTEIN g | CARBOHYDRATE g | FIBRE g |
|---|---|---|---|---|---|---|
| 66 | 283 | Trace | Trace | 0 | 17 | 0.4 |
| 94 | 397 | 4 | Trace | 0 | 16 | 0.3 |
| 62 | 266 | Trace | Trace | 0 | 16 | 0.3 |
| 51 | 219 | Trace | Trace | 0 | 13 | 0.3 |
| 42 | 179 | Trace | Trace | 0 | 10 | 0.4 |
| | | | | | | |
| 108 | 445 | 11 | 3.7 | 1 | 1 | Trace |
| 58 | 239 | 6 | 1.2 | 1 | 1 | 1.1 |
| 56 | 234 | 4 | 0.5 | 2 | 3 | 0.7 |
| 227 | 935 | 24 | 1.8 | 1 | 2 | Trace |
| 30 | 124 | 2 | 1.3 | 2 | 1 | 0.1 |
| | | | | | | |
| 114 | 472 | 12 | 6.2 | 1 | 2 | 0 |
| 10 | 42 | 0 | 0 | 0 | 2 | 0 |
| 69 | 285 | 7 | 0.6 | 0 | 1 | 0 |
| 11 | 45 | 1 | 0.1 | 0 | 1 | Trace |
| 97 | 399 | 11 | 1.1 | 0 | 0 | Trace |
| 97 | 401 | 9 | 0.9 | 0 | 4 | 0.1 |
| 59 | 243 | 5 | 0.5 | 0 | 4 | Trace |
| 88 | 363 | 8 | 0.8 | 1 | 3 | Trace |
| | | | | | | |
| 207 | 853 | 23 | 3.3 | 0 | 1 | 0 |
| 237 | 974 | 26 | 3.8 | 1 | 0 | Trace |
| 217 | 894 | 24 | 3.5 | 1 | 0 | 0 |
| 86 | 356 | 8 | 1.1 | 0 | 2 | 0 |

| MAYONNAISE AND SALAD CREAM | AVERAGE PORTION g |
|---|---|
| Salad cream | 20 |
| Salad cream, reduced-calorie | 20 |

## PICKLES

| | |
|---|---|
| Gherkins, pickled | 25 |
| Onions, pickled | 30 |
| Piccalilli | 40 |
| Pickle, chilli, oily | 15 |
| Pickle, chow chow, sour | 15 |
| Pickle, chow chow, sweet | 15 |
| Pickle, lime, oily | 15 |
| Pickle, mango, oily | 15 |
| Pickle, mixed vegetables | 15 |
| Pickle, sweet | 15 |

## COOKING SAUCES

| | |
|---|---|
| Barbecue sauce | 25 |
| Black bean sauce | 20 |
| Chilli sauce | 25 |
| Cook-in-sauces, canned, different flavours | 150 |
| Curry sauce, canned | 150 |
| Oyster sauce | 15 |
| Sauce, curry, sweet | 150 |
| Sauce, curry, tomato and onion | 150 |
| Soy sauce, dark, thick | 5 |
| Soy sauce, light, thin | 5 |
| Tomato sauce | 90 |
| Pasta sauce, tomato based | 170 |

| ENERGY kcal | ENERGY kJ | FAT g | SATURATED FAT g | PROTEIN g | CARBOHYDRATE g | FIBRE g |
|---|---|---|---|---|---|---|
| 70 | 288 | 6 | 0.8 | 0 | 3 | 0 |
| 39 | 161 | 3 | 0.5 | 0 | 2 | 0 |
| 4 | 15 | Trace | Trace | 0 | 1 | 0.3 |
| 7 | 30 | Trace | Trace | 0 | 1 | 0.4 |
| 34 | 144 | 0 | 0 | 0 | 7 | 0.4 |
| 41 | 168 | 4 | Trace | 0 | 1 | 0.2 |
| 4 | 18 | 0 | 0 | 0 | 1 | 0.2 |
| 17 | 73 | 0 | 0 | 0 | 4 | 0.2 |
| 27 | 111 | 2 | Trace | 0 | 1 | 0.2 |
| 27 | 110 | 2 | Trace | 0 | 1 | 0.2 |
| 3 | 14 | 0 | 0 | 0 | 1 | 0.2 |
| 21 | 91 | 0 | Trace | 0 | 5 | 0.2 |
| 23 | 99 | 0 | 0 | 0 | 6 | 0.1 |
| 19 | 79 | 0 | 0 | 1 | 2 | 0.4 |
| 20 | 84 | Trace | Trace | 0 | 4 | 0.3 |
| 65 | 272 | 4 | 0.2 | 2 | 12 | Trace |
| 117 | 486 | 8 | 0.4 | 2 | 11 | Trace |
| 12 | 51 | 0 | Trace | 1 | 3 | Trace |
| 137 | 570 | 8 | 2.3 | 2 | 14 | 2.1 |
| 297 | 1229 | 29 | 3 | 3 | 9 | 1.7 |
| 3 | 13 | 0 | 0 | 0 | 0 | 00 |
| 3 | 13 | 0 | 0 | 0 | 0 | 0 |
| 80 | 337 | 5 | 1.6 | 2 | 8 | 1.3 |
| 80 | 340 | 3 | 0,3 | 3 | 12 | 2.5 |

| CUSTARDS | AVERAGE PORTION g |
|---|---|
| Crème caramel | 90 |
| Custard, canned, ready-to-serve | 120 |
| Custard, canned, ready-to-serve, low-fat | 120 |
| Custard, chilled, ready-to-serve | 120 |
| Custard, confectioners' | 150 |
| Custard, made with semi-skimmed milk | 150 |
| Custard, made with whole milk | 120 |

| ENERGY kcal | ENERGY kJ | FAT g | SATURATED FAT g | PROTEIN g | CARBOHYDRATE g | FIBRE g |
|---|---|---|---|---|---|---|
| 98 | 416 | 1 | Trace | 3 | 19 | Trace |
| 118 | 497 | 3 | 2.3 | 3 | 20 | 0.0 |
| | | | | | | |
| 93 | 395 | 2 | 0.0 | 3 | 18 | 0.0 |
| 135 | 569 | 6 | 4.4 | 3 | 18 | 0.0 |
| 255 | 1077 | 9 | 4.1 | 10 | 37 | 0.3 |
| | | | | | | |
| 141 | 605 | 3 | 1.8 | 6 | 25 | Trace |
| 140 | 594 | 5 | 3.4 | 4 | 20 | Trace |

| PASTRY | AVERAGE PORTION g |
|---|---|
| Cheese | 100 |
| Choux | 100 |
| Flaky | 100 |
| Shortcrust | 100 |
| Wholemeal | 100 |

## PASTRY DISHES

| | |
|---|---|
| Beef pie, shop bought | 141 |
| Chicken and mushroom pie, single crust | 100 |
| Chicken pie, individual, baked | 130 |
| Cornish pasty | 155 |
| Cornish pasty, shop bought | 155 |
| Lamb samosa, baked | 70 |
| Lamb samosa, deep-fried | 70 |
| Pasty, vegetable | 155 |
| Pasty, vegetable, wholemeal | 155 |
| Pork and egg pie | 60 |
| Pork pie | 60 |
| Pork pie, mini | 50 |
| Quiche, broccoli | 140 |
| Quiche, broccoli, wholemeal | 140 |
| Quiche, cauliflower cheese | 140 |
| Quiche, cauliflower cheese, wholemeal | 140 |
| Quiche, cheese and egg | 140 |
| Quiche, cheese and egg, wholemeal | 140 |
| Quiche, cheese and mushroom | 140 |
| Quiche, cheese and mushroom, wholemeal | 140 |
| Quiche, cheese, onion and potato | 140 |
| Quiche, cheese, onion and potato, wholemeal | 140 |
| Quiche, mushroom | 140 |

Unless otherwise specified, all pastry dishes are homemade.

| ENERGY kcal | ENERGY kJ | FAT g | SATURATED FAT g | PROTEIN g | CARBOHYDRATE g | FIBRE g |
|---|---|---|---|---|---|---|
| 500 | 2083 | 34 | 15.3 | 13 | 37 | 1.5 |
| 325 | 1355 | 20 | 15 | 9 | 30 | 1.2 |
| 560 | 2332 | 41 | 14.7 | 6 | 46 | 1.8 |
| 521 | 2174 | 32 | 11.7 | 7 | 54 | 2.2 |
| 499 | 2080 | 33 | 11.8 | 9 | 45 | 6.3 |
| | | | | | | |
| 437 | 1826 | 24 | 11.8 | 12 | 38 | 0.7 |
| | | | | | | |
| 200 | 836 | 10 | 4.5 | 13 | 14 | 0.6 |
| 374 | 1563 | 21 | 9.1 | 12 | 32 | 1 |
| 456 | 1905 | 28 | 9.8 | 10 | 43 | 2.6 |
| 414 | 1731 | 25 | 9.1 | 10 | 39 | 1.4 |
| 187 | 781 | 10 | 2.5 | 8 | 16 | 1.2 |
| 265 | 1097 | 22 | 3.3 | 6 | 12 | 0.8 |
| 425 | 1783 | 23 | 5.7 | 6 | 52 | 2.9 |
| 406 | 1702 | 24 | 5.7 | 8 | 43 | 6.4 |
| 178 | 740 | 13 | 4.4 | 6 | 10 | 0.5 |
| 228 | 947 | 18 | 6.8 | 6 | 11 | 0.5 |
| 196 | 815 | 14 | 5.7 | 5 | 13 | 0.5 |
| 349 | 1455 | 21 | 8.3 | 12 | 30 | 1.7 |
| 337 | 1408 | 21 | 8.3 | 13 | 25 | 3.8 |
| 277 | 1156 | 18 | 7.1 | 7 | 24 | 1.5 |
| 269 | 1121 | 18 | 7.1 | 8 | 20 | 3.1 |
| 440 | 1834 | 31 | 14.4 | 18 | 24 | 0.8 |
| 431 | 1796 | 31 | 14.6 | 18 | 20 | 2.7 |
| 396 | 1655 | 26 | 10.8 | 15 | 26 | 1.3 |
| | | | | | | |
| 388 | 1616 | 27 | 10.8 | 16 | 22 | 3.1 |
| 480 | 2005 | 33 | 16 | 18 | 28 | 1.4 |
| | | | | | | |
| 472 | 1966 | 34 | 16.1 | 19 | 25 | 3.1 |
| 398 | 1659 | 27 | 12.2 | 14 | 26 | 1.3 |

## PASTRY DISHES

| | AVERAGE PORTION g |
|---|---|
| Quiche, mushroom, wholemeal | 140 |
| Quiche, spinach | 140 |
| Quiche, spinach, wholemeal | 140 |
| Quiche, vegetable | 140 |
| Quiche, vegetable, wholemeal | 140 |
| Sausage rolls, flaky pastry | 60 |
| Sausage rolls, shortcrust pastry | 60 |
| Steak and kidney pie, double crust | 120 |
| Steak and kidney pie, shop bought | 141 |

Unless otherwise specified, all pastry dishes are homemade.

| ENERGY kcal | ENERGY kJ | FAT g | SATURATED FAT g | PROTEIN g | CARBOHYDRATE g | FIBRE g |
|---|---|---|---|---|---|---|
| 388 | 1618 | 28 | 12.2 | 15 | 21 | 3.1 |
| 287 | 1203 | 18 | 5.6 | 14 | 18 | 2 |
| 281 | 1176 | 18 | 5.6 | 15 | 16 | 3.2 |
| 295 | 1238 | 18 | 6 | 7 | 28 | 2.1 |
| 286 | 1197 | 18 | 6 | 8 | 24 | 3.9 |
| 238 | 991 | 17 | 6.5 | 6 | 15 | 0.8 |
| 229 | 953 | 16 | 5.8 | 6 | 17 | 0.9 |
| 406 | 1694 | 26 | 9.7 | 16 | 27 | 1.1 |
| 437 | 1826 | 24 | 11.8 | 12 | 38 | 0.7 |

| MILK-BASED PUDDINGS AND DESSERTS | AVERAGE PORTION g |
|---|---|
| Blancmange | 150 |
| Fruit fool | 120 |
| Fruit fool, low-fat | 120 |
| Milk pudding, made with semi-skimmed milk | 200 |
| Milk pudding, made with whole milk | 200 |
| Rice desserts, individual, with fruit | 135 |
| Rice pudding, canned | 200 |
| Tiramisu | 90 |
| Trifle, chocolate | 113 |
| Trifle, fruit | 113 |

| CHEESECAKES | |
|---|---|
| Chocolate | 120 |
| Frozen | 90 |
| Fruit, individual | 90 |
| Fruit, large | 120 |

| OTHER DESSERTS | |
|---|---|
| Christmas pudding | 100 |
| Crumble, fruit | 170 |
| Jelly, made with water | 115 |
| Pavlova, chocolate | 100 |
| Pavlova, fruit | 100 |
| Profiteroles with chocolate sauce | 155 |
| Strudel, fruit | 115 |

| MOUSSE | |
|---|---|
| Chocolate, individual | 60 |
| Chocolate | 60 |
| Fruit | 60 |

| ENERGY kcal | ENERGY kJ | FAT g | SATURATED FAT g | PROTEIN g | CARBOHYDRATE g | FIBRE g |
| --- | --- | --- | --- | --- | --- | --- |
| 171 | 720 | 6 | 3.4 | 5 | 27 | Trace |
| 213 | 890 | 13 | 8.8 | 3 | 22 | 0.5 |
| 97 | 405 | 6 | 0.0 | 4 | 8 | 0.5l |
| 214 | 914 | 4 | 2.2 | 8 | 40 | 0.2 |
| 258 | 1086 | 9 | 5.4 | 8 | 40 | 0.2 |
| 153 | 648 | 3 | 2.0 | 4 | 29 | 0.4 |
| 178 | 748 | 3 | 3.2 | 7 | 28 | 0.4 |
| 220 | 919 | 13 | 7.7 | 4 | 24 | 0.4 |
| 233 | 971 | 17 | 10.7 | 5 | 15 | 1.4 |
| 161 | 672 | 10 | 6.3 | 3 | 15 | 2.4 |
| 415 | 1731 | 28 | 14.4 | 6 | 37 | 0.8 |
| 218 | 915 | 10 | 5 | 5 | 30 | 0.8 |
| 238 | 1000 | 11 | 6.8 | 5 | 31 | 0.9 |
| 353 | 1477 | 19 | 11.8 | 5 | 42 | 1.0 |
| 291 | 1227 | 10 | 4.5 | 5 | 50 | 1.3 |
| 373 | 1571 | 14 | 6.7 | 4 | 61 | 2.2 |
| 70 | 299 | 0 | 0 | 1 | 17 | 0 |
| 370 | 1552 | 20 | 10.7 | 4 | 47 | 0.3 |
| 288 | 1210 | 13 | 7.1 | 3 | 42 | 0.3 |
| 535 | 2226 | 40 | 21.7 | 9 | 38 | 1.1 |
| 279 | 1167 | 16 | 6.0 | 3 | 33 | 1.2 |
| 83 | 352 | 4 | 2.7 | 2 | 12 | 0.1 |
| 73 | 310 | 2 | 1.5 | 3 | 11 | 0.1 |
| 82 | 345 | 3 | 2 | 3 | 11 | 0.1 |

DESSERTS &
ICE CREAMS

| PIES | AVERAGE PORTION g |
|---|---|
| Apple pie, deep filled, double crust | 110 |
| Apple pie, double crust | 110 |
| Banoffee pie | 150 |
| Lemon meringue pie | 150 |
| Mince pies, individual | 55 |
| Mississippi mud pie | 150 |

## ICE CREAM AND FROZEN DESSERTS

| | |
|---|---|
| Arctic roll | 50 |
| Banana split | 100 |
| Chocolate-covered ice cream bar | 51 |
| Chocolate nut sundae | 60 |
| Frozen ice cream dessert, chocolate | 60 |
| Frozen ice cream dessert, plain | 60 |
| Ice cream, chocolate | 75 |
| Ice cream, dairy-free | 75 |
| Ice cream, fruit | 75 |
| Ice cream, luxury, vanilla | 75 |
| Ice cream, soya | 75 |
| Ice cream, vanilla | 75 |
| Ice cream, virtually fat free | 75 |
| Ice cream bar, chocolate flavoured coating | 48 |
| Ice cream cone, chocolate/mint/nuts | 73 |
| Ice cream cone, strawberry | 81 |
| Knickerbocker glory | 100 |
| Kulfi | 80 |
| Lolly, fruit | 73 |
| Lolly, ice cream, with fruit coating | 73 |
| Peach melba | 60 |
| Sorbet, fruit | 75 |

| ENERGY kcal | ENERGY kJ | FAT g | SATURATED FAT g | PROTEIN g | CARBOHYDRATE g | FIBRE g |
|---|---|---|---|---|---|---|
| 281 | 1183 | 12 | 3.8 | 4 | 42 | 1.1 |
| 269 | 1129 | 14 | 4.5 | 4 | 33 | 1.1 |
| 478 | 1997 | 30 | 15.0 | 6 | 49 | 3.8 |
| 377 | 1590 | 13 | 4.6 | 4 | 65 | 0.7 |
| 233 | 975 | 11 | 4.1 | 2 | 32 | 1.2 |
| 478 | 1997 | 30 | 15.0 | 6 | 49 | 3.8 |
| | | | | | | |
| 100 | 424 | 3 | 1.5 | 2 | 17 | Trace |
| 182 | 761 | 11 | 6 | 2 | 19 | 0.6 |
| 163 | 679 | 2 | 7.7 | 3 | 12 | 0 |
| 167 | 699 | 9 | 5 | 2 | 21 | 0.1 |
| 150 | 627 | 11 | 8.5 | 2 | 13 | 0.0 |
| 136 | 568 | 9 | 6.7 | 2 | 14 | Trace |
| 156 | 653 | 8 | 5.2 | 3 | 19 | 0.0 |
| 156 | 654 | 9 | 2.8 | 2 | 17 | 0.1 |
| 119 | 499 | 5 | 3.4 | 2 | 17 | 0.2 |
| 161 | 670 | 11 | 6.8 | 3 | 13 | 0.0 |
| 156 | 654 | 9 | 2.8 | 2 | 17 | 0.1 |
| 115 | 480 | 6 | 3.6 | 2 | 14 | 0.0 |
| 76 | 324 | 1 | Trace | 3 | 15 | 0.0 |
| | | | | | | |
| 142 | 590 | 10 | 8.8 | 2 | 11 | 0.0 |
| 207 | 867 | 13 | 9.6 | 3 | 21 | 0.2 |
| 201 | 844 | 10 | 7.1 | 3 | 28 | 0.2 |
| 112 | 473 | 5 | 2.9 | 2 | 16 | 0.2 |
| 339 | 1405 | 32 | 18.2 | 4 | 9 | 0.5 |
| 56 | 234 | 1 | 0.1 | 0 | 14 | 0.1 |
| 78 | 326 | 2 | 1 | 1 | 15 | 0.1 |
| 98 | 411 | 6 | 3.8 | 1 | 10 | 0.2 |
| 98 | 422 | Trace | Trace | 1 | 26 | 0 |

| CONFECTIONERY | AVERAGE PORTION g |
|---|---|
| Boiled sweets | 7 |
| Bounty® bar | 57 |
| Chewy sweets | 3 |
| Chocolate, cooking | 50 |
| Chocolate, diabetic | 50 |
| Chocolate, fancy and filled | 8 |
| Chocolate, milk | 54 |
| Chocolate, plain | 50 |
| Chocolate, white | 50 |
| Chocolate-covered bar with fruit/nut | 34 |
| Chocolate-covered bar with wafer/biscuit | 34 |
| Chocolate-covered biscuit fingers | 28 |
| Chocolate-covered caramels | 5 |
| Chocolate-covered wafer biscuits | 22 |
| Creme eggs® | 39 |
| Fruit gums/jellies | 2 |
| Fudge | 11 |
| Liquorice allsorts | 7 |
| Mars® bar | 65 |
| Marshmallows | 5 |
| Milky Way® | 26 |
| Nougat | 70 |
| Pastilles | 3 |
| Peanut brittle | 58 |
| Peppermint creams | 6 |
| Peppermints | 6 |
| Sherbert sweets | 5 |
| Smartie®-type sweets | 15 |
| Toffees, mixed | 8 |
| Truffles, mocha | 7 |
| Truffles, rum | 7 |
| Turkish delight, with nuts | 15 |
| Turkish delight, without nuts | 15 |

| ENERGY kcal | ENERGY kJ | FAT g | SATURATED FAT g | PROTEIN g | CARBOHYDRATE g | FIBRE g |
|---|---|---|---|---|---|---|
| 23 | 98 | Trace | 0 | Trace | 6 | 0 |
| 270 | 1129 | 15 | 12.1 | 3 | 33 | 1.4 |
| 11 | 48 | 1 | 0.1 | 0 | 3 | 0 |
| 275 | 1147 | 17 | 14 | 2 | 29 | 0.6 |
| 224 | 934 | 15 | 9.1 | 5 | 19 | 0.6 |
| 36 | 150 | 2 | 0.9 | 0 | 5 | 0.1 |
| 281 | 1176 | 17 | 9.9 | 4 | 31 | 0.4 |
| 255 | 1069 | 14 | 8.4 | 3 | 32 | 1.3 |
| 265 | 1106 | 15 | 9.2 | 4 | 29 | 0 |
| 170 | 711 | 9 | 4.6 | 3 | 20 | 1.3 |
| 170 | 711 | 9 | 4.6 | 3 | 20 | 1.3 |
| 134 | 564 | 7 | 3.4 | 2 | 18 | 0.3 |
| 23 | 98 | 1 | 0.5 | 0 | 3 | 0 |
| 110 | 462 | 6 | 3.8 | 2 | 14 | 0.2 |
| 163 | 681 | 6 | 1.8 | 2 | 28 | 0.5 |
| 6 | 28 | 0 | 0 | 0 | 2 | Trace |
| 49 | 205 | 2 | 1 | 0 | 9 | 0 |
| 24 | 104 | 1 | 0.3 | 0 | 5 | 0.1 |
| 287 | 1204 | 12 | 6.5 | 3 | 43 | 0.7 |
| 16 | 70 | 0 | 0 | 0 | 4 | 0 |
| 103 | 435 | 4 | 2.2 | 1 | 16 | 0.2 |
| 269 | 1138 | 6 | 0.8 | 3 | 54 | 0.6 |
| 8 | 32 | 0 | 0 | 0 | 2 | 0 |
| 280 | 1178 | 11 | 3.1 | 5 | 43 | 1.2 |
| 22 | 95 | Trace | 0 | 0 | 6 | Trace |
| 24 | 101 | 0 | 0 | 0 | 6 | 0 |
| 18 | 76 | 0 | 0 | 0 | 5 | Trace |
| 68 | 288 | 3 | 1.6 | 1 | 11 | 0.2 |
| 34 | 143 | 1 | 0.8 | 0 | 5 | 0 |
| 34 | 143 | 2 | 1.1 | 0 | 4 | 0.1 |
| 36 | 152 | 2 | 1.4 | 0 | 3 | 0.1 |
| 52 | 219 | 0 | 0 | 1 | 12 | 0 |
| 44 | 189 | 0 | 0 | 0 | 12 | 0 |

| COLD BEVERAGES<br>CARBONATED DRINKS | AVERAGE PORTION ml |
|---|---|
| Cola | 160 |
| Cola, diet | 160 |
| Ginger ale, dry | 160 |
| Ginger ale, dry, diet | 160 |
| Lemonade | 160 |
| Lemonade, diet | 160 |
| Lucozade | 160 |
| Orangeade | 160 |
| Orangeade, diet | 160 |
| Root beer | 160 |
| Soda, cream | 160 |
| Tonic water | 160 |

| FRUIT JUICES | |
|---|---|
| Apple, unsweetened | 160 |
| Carrot | 160 |
| Grape, unsweetened | 160 |
| Grapefruit, unsweetened | 160 |
| Lemon, fresh | 10 |
| Lime, fresh | 10 |
| Mango, canned | 160 |
| Orange, freshly squeezed | 160 |
| Orange, unsweetened | 160 |
| Passion fruit | 160 |
| Pineapple, unsweetened | 160 |
| Pomegranate, fresh | 160 |
| Prune | 160 |
| Tomato | 160 |

| ENERGY kcal | ENERGY kJ | FAT g | SATURATED FAT g | PROTEIN g | CARBOHYDRATE g | FIBRE g |
|---|---|---|---|---|---|---|
| 66 | 278 | 0 | 0 | Trace | 17 | 0 |
| Trace | Trace | 0 | 0 | 0 | 0 | 0 |
| 24 | 99 | 0 | 0 | 0 | 6 | 0 |
| 2 | 6 | 0 | 0 | 0 | 0.4 | 0 |
| 35 | 149 | 0 | 0 | Trace | 9 | 0 |
| Trace | Trace | 0 | 0 | 0 | 0 | 0 |
| 96 | 410 | 0 | 0 | Trace | 26 | 0 |
| 113 | 474 | 0 | 0 | 0 | 27 | 0 |
| 1 | 4 | 0 | 0 | 0 | 0.4 | 0 |
| 66 | 275 | 0 | 0 | 0 | 17 | 0 |
| 82 | 344 | 0 | 0 | 0 | 21 | 0 |
| 53 | 226 | 0 | 0 | 0 | 14 | 0 |
| 61 | 262 | Trace | Trace | 0 | 16 | Trace |
| 38 | 165 | Trace | Trace | 1 | 9 | 0.2 |
| 74 | 314 | Trace | Trace | 0 | 19 | 0 |
| 53 | 224 | Trace | Trace | 1 | 13 | Trace |
| 1 | 3 | Trace | Trace | 0 | 0 | 0 |
| 1 | 4 | Trace | Trace | 0 | 0 | 0 |
| 62 | 266 | Trace | Trace | 0 | 16 | Trace |
| 53 | 224 | Trace | Trace | 1 | 13 | 0.2 |
| 58 | 245 | Trace | Trace | 1 | 14 | 0.2 |
| 75 | 302 | Trace | Trace | 1 | 17 | Trace |
| 66 | 283 | Trace | Trace | 0 | 17 | Trace |
| 70 | 302 | Trace | Trace | 0 | 19 | Trace |
| 91 | 389 | Trace | Trace | 1 | 23 | Trace |
| 22 | 99 | Trace | Trace | 1 | 5 | 1 |

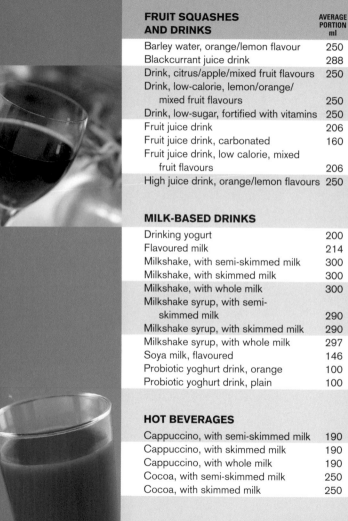

| FRUIT SQUASHES AND DRINKS | AVERAGE PORTION ml |
|---|---|
| Barley water, orange/lemon flavour | 250 |
| Blackcurrant juice drink | 288 |
| Drink, citrus/apple/mixed fruit flavours | 250 |
| Drink, low-calorie, lemon/orange/ mixed fruit flavours | 250 |
| Drink, low-sugar, fortified with vitamins | 250 |
| Fruit juice drink | 206 |
| Fruit juice drink, carbonated | 160 |
| Fruit juice drink, low calorie, mixed fruit flavours | 206 |
| High juice drink, orange/lemon flavours | 250 |

| MILK-BASED DRINKS | |
|---|---|
| Drinking yogurt | 200 |
| Flavoured milk | 214 |
| Milkshake, with semi-skimmed milk | 300 |
| Milkshake, with skimmed milk | 300 |
| Milkshake, with whole milk | 300 |
| Milkshake syrup, with semi- skimmed milk | 290 |
| Milkshake syrup, with skimmed milk | 290 |
| Milkshake syrup, with whole milk | 297 |
| Soya milk, flavoured | 146 |
| Probiotic yoghurt drink, orange | 100 |
| Probiotic yoghurt drink, plain | 100 |

| HOT BEVERAGES | |
|---|---|
| Cappuccino, with semi-skimmed milk | 190 |
| Cappuccino, with skimmed milk | 190 |
| Cappuccino, with whole milk | 190 |
| Cocoa, with semi-skimmed milk | 250 |
| Cocoa, with skimmed milk | 250 |

| ENERGY kcal | ENERGY kJ | FAT g | SATURATED FAT g | PROTEIN g | CARBOHYDRATE g | FIBRE g |
|---|---|---|---|---|---|---|
| 35 | 150 | 0 | 0 | 0 | 9 | 0 |
| 86 | 372 | 0 | 0 | Trace | 23 | 0 |
| 48 | 200 | 0 | 0 | Trace | 13 | 0 |
|  |  |  |  |  |  |  |
| 3 | 8 | 0 | 0 | Trace | 1 | 0 |
| 10 | 43 | 0 | 0 | Trace | 3 | 0 |
| 76 | 328 | Trace | Trace | 0 | 20 | Trace |
| 62 | 264 | Trace | Trace | Trace | 16 | Trace |
|  |  |  |  |  |  |  |
| 21 | 89 | Trace | Trace | 0 | 5 | Trace |
| 63 | 268 | 0 | 0 | 0 | 16 | 0 |
|  |  |  |  |  |  |  |
| 124 | 526 | Trace | Trace | 6 | 26 | Trace |
| 146 | 614 | 3 | 1.9 | 8 | 23 | 0 |
| 207 | 882 | 5 | 3 | 10 | 34 | Trace |
| 171 | 726 | 1 | 0.3 | 10 | 34 | 0 |
| 261 | 1104 | 11 | 7.2 | 9 | 33 | Trace |
|  |  |  |  |  |  |  |
| 171 | 725 | 4 | 2.6 | 8 | 27 | 0 |
| 136 | 576 | 1 | 0.2 | 9 | 27 | 0 |
| 223 | 936 | 10 | 6.2 | 8 | 27 | 0 |
| 58 | 245 | 2 | 0.3 | 4 | 5 | Trace |
| 67 | 279 | 0.9 | 0.6 | 1.5 | 13.4 | 1.3 |
| 68 | 284 | 1 | 0.7 | 1.7 | 13.1 | 1.4 |
|  |  |  |  |  |  |  |
| 46 | 193 | 2 | 1 | 3 | 5 | 0 |
| 33 | 141 | 0 | 0.1 | 3 | 5 | 0 |
| 65 | 269 | 4 | 2.3 | 3 | 5 | 0 |
| 143 | 608 | 5 | 3 | 9 | 18 | 0.5 |
| 110 | 475 | 1 | 0.8 | 9 | 18 | 0.5 |

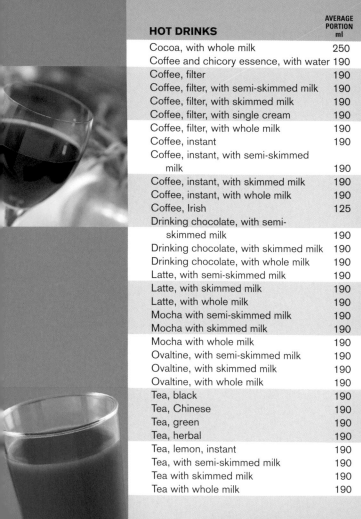

| HOT DRINKS | AVERAGE PORTION ml |
|---|---|
| Cocoa, with whole milk | 250 |
| Coffee and chicory essence, with water | 190 |
| Coffee, filter | 190 |
| Coffee, filter, with semi-skimmed milk | 190 |
| Coffee, filter, with skimmed milk | 190 |
| Coffee, filter, with single cream | 190 |
| Coffee, filter, with whole milk | 190 |
| Coffee, instant | 190 |
| Coffee, instant, with semi-skimmed milk | 190 |
| Coffee, instant, with skimmed milk | 190 |
| Coffee, instant, with whole milk | 190 |
| Coffee, Irish | 125 |
| Drinking chocolate, with semi-skimmed milk | 190 |
| Drinking chocolate, with skimmed milk | 190 |
| Drinking chocolate, with whole milk | 190 |
| Latte, with semi-skimmed milk | 190 |
| Latte, with skimmed milk | 190 |
| Latte, with whole milk | 190 |
| Mocha with semi-skimmed milk | 190 |
| Mocha with skimmed milk | 190 |
| Mocha with whole milk | 190 |
| Ovaltine, with semi-skimmed milk | 190 |
| Ovaltine, with skimmed milk | 190 |
| Ovaltine, with whole milk | 190 |
| Tea, black | 190 |
| Tea, Chinese | 190 |
| Tea, green | 190 |
| Tea, herbal | 190 |
| Tea, lemon, instant | 190 |
| Tea, with semi-skimmed milk | 190 |
| Tea with skimmed milk | 190 |
| Tea with whole milk | 190 |

| ENERGY kcal | ENERGY kJ | FAT g | SATURATED FAT g | PROTEIN g | CARBOHYDRATE g | FIBRE g |
|---|---|---|---|---|---|---|
| 190 | 800 | 10 | 6.5 | 9 | 17 | 0.5 |
| 17 | 76 | Trace | 0 | 0 | 5 | 0 |
| 4 | 15 | Trace | Trace | 0 | 1 | 0 |
| 13 | 55 | 1 | 0.2 | 1 | 1 | 0 |
| 11 | 43 | 0 | 0 | 1 | 1 | 0 |
| 27 | 106 | 2 | 1.3 | 1 | 1 | 0 |
| 13 | 59 | 1 | 0.6 | 1 | 1 | 0 |
| Trace | 4 | Trace | 0 | 0 | Trace | 0 |
| 13 | 55 | 1 | 0.2 | 1 | 1 | 0 |
| 8 | 39 | 0 | 0 | 1 | 1 | 0 |
| 15 | 65 | 1 | 0.6 | 1 | 1 | 0 |
| 105 | 433 | 10 | 6.1 | 1 | 4 | 0 |
| 135 | 578 | 4 | 2.3 | 7 | 21 | Trace |
| 112 | 481 | 1 | 0.6 | 7 | 21 | Trace |
| 171 | 716 | 8 | 4.8 | 6 | 20 | Trace |
| 60 | 252 | 2 | 1.3 | 4 | 7 | 0 |
| 33 | 141 | 1 | 0.1 | 3 | 5 | 0 |
| 85 | 353 | 5 | 3 | 4 | 6 | 0 |
| 96 | 405 | 5 | 3.1 | 4 | 9 | 0.1 |
| 81 | 339 | 3 | 2 | 4 | 9 | 0.1 |
| 120 | 500 | 7 | 4.8 | 4 | 9 | 0.1 |
| 150 | 642 | 3 | 1.9 | 7 | 25 | Trace |
| 129 | 549 | 1 | 0.2 | 7 | 25 | Trace |
| 184 | 779 | 7 | 4.6 | 7 | 25 | Trace |
| Trace | 4 | Trace | Trace | 0 | Trace | 0 |
| 2 | 10 | 0 | 0 | 0 | 0 | 0 |
| Trace | Trace | 0 | 0 | 0 | Trace | 0 |
| 2 | 25 | Trace | Trace | 0 | 0 | 0 |
| 15 | 65 | 0 | 0 | 0 | 4 | 0 |
| 13 | 53 | 1 | 0.2 | 1 | 1 | 0 |
| 8 | 36 | 0 | 0 | 1 | 1 | 0 |
| 15 | 61 | 1 | 0.6 | 1 | 1 | 0 |

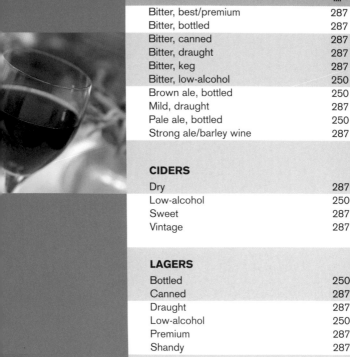

| **BEERS** | **AVERAGE PORTION ml** |
|---|---|
| Bitter, best/premium | 287 |
| Bitter, bottled | 287 |
| Bitter, canned | 287 |
| Bitter, draught | 287 |
| Bitter, keg | 287 |
| Bitter, low-alcohol | 250 |
| Brown ale, bottled | 250 |
| Mild, draught | 287 |
| Pale ale, bottled | 250 |
| Strong ale/barley wine | 287 |

| **CIDERS** | |
|---|---|
| Dry | 287 |
| Low-alcohol | 250 |
| Sweet | 287 |
| Vintage | 287 |

| **LAGERS** | |
|---|---|
| Bottled | 250 |
| Canned | 287 |
| Draught | 287 |
| Low-alcohol | 250 |
| Premium | 287 |
| Shandy | 287 |

| ENERGY kcal | ENERGY kJ | FAT g | SATURATED FAT g | PROTEIN g | CARBOHYDRATE g | FIBRE g |
|---|---|---|---|---|---|---|
| 95 | 399 | Trace | Trace | 1 | 6 | Trace |
| 86 | 356 | Trace | Trace | 1 | 6 | Trace |
| 92 | 379 | Trace | Trace | 1 | 7 | 0 |
| 92 | 379 | Trace | Trace | 1 | 7 | 0 |
| 89 | 370 | Trace | Trace | 1 | 7 | 0 |
| 33 | 135 | 0 | 0 | 1 | 5 | Trace |
| 75 | 315 | Trace | Trace | 1 | 8 | Trace |
| 69 | 293 | Trace | Trace | 1 | 5 | Trace |
| 70 | 295 | Trace | Trace | 1 | 5 | Trace |
| 189 | 789 | Trace | Trace | 2 | 18 | Trace |
| | | | | | | |
| | | | | | | |
| 103 | 436 | 0 | 0 | Trace | 7 | 0 |
| 43 | 185 | 0 | 0 | Trace | 9 | 0 |
| 121 | 505 | 0 | 0 | Trace | 12 | 0 |
| 290 | 1208 | 0 | 0 | Trace | 21 | 0 |
| | | | | | | |
| | | | | | | |
| 73 | 300 | Trace | Trace | 1 | 4 | 0 |
| 83 | 347 | Trace | Trace | 1 | Trace | Trace |
| 83 | 347 | Trace | Trace | 1 | Trace | Trace |
| 25 | 103 | Trace | Trace | 1 | 4 | Trace |
| 169 | 700 | Trace | Trace | 1 | 7 | Trace |
| 32 | 138 | 0 | 0 | Trace | 9 | Trace |

| LIQUEURS | AVERAGE PORTION ml |
|---|---|
| Advocaat | 25 |
| Cherry Brandy | 25 |
| Coîntreau | 25 |
| Cream liqueurs | 25 |
| Crème de Menthe | 25 |
| Curaçao | 25 |
| Drambuie | 25 |
| Egg nog | 160 |
| Grand Marnier | 25 |
| Pernod | 25 |
| Southern Comfort | 25 |
| Tia Maria | 25 |

| FORTIFIED WINES | |
|---|---|
| Port | 50 |
| Sherry, dry | 50 |
| Sherry, medium | 50 |
| Sherry, sweet | 50 |
| Tonic wine | 125 |
| Vermouth, dry | 48 |
| Vermouth, sweet | 48 |

| SPIRITS, 40% VOLUME | |
|---|---|
| Brandy | 25 |
| Gin | 25 |
| Rum | 25 |
| Vodka | 25 |
| Whisky | 25 |

| ENERGY kcal | ENERGY kJ | FAT g | SATURATED FAT g | PROTEIN g | CARBOHYDRATE g | FIBRE g |
|---|---|---|---|---|---|---|
| 65 | 273 | 2 | 0.5 | 1 | 7 | 0 |
| 66 | 275 | 0 | 0 | Trace | 8 | 0 |
| 79 | 328 | 0 | 0 | Trace | 6 | 0 |
| 81 | 338 | 4 | 0 | Trace | 6 | 0 |
| 66 | 275 | 0 | 0 | Trace | 8 | 0 |
| 78 | 326 | 0 | 0 | Trace | 7 | 0 |
| 79 | 328 | 0 | 0 | Trace | 6 | 0 |
| 182 | 763 | 7 | 3.4 | 6 | 16 | 0 |
| 79 | 328 | 0 | 0 | Trace | 6 | 0 |
| 79 | 328 | 0 | 0 | Trace | 6 | 0 |
| 79 | 328 | 0 | 0 | Trace | 6 | 0 |
| 66 | 275 | 0 | 0 | Trace | 8 | 0 |
| | | | | | | |
| 79 | 328 | 0 | 0 | 0 | 6 | 0 |
| 58 | 241 | 0 | 0 | 0 | 1 | 0 |
| 58 | 241 | 0 | 0 | 0 | 3 | 0 |
| 68 | 284 | 0 | 0 | 0 | 3 | 0 |
| 159 | 665 | 0 | 0 | Trace | 15 | 0 |
| 52 | 217 | 0 | 0 | 0 | 1 | 0 |
| 72 | 303 | 0 | 0 | Trace | 8 | 0 |
| | | | | | | |
| 52 | 215 | 0 | 0 | Trace | Trace | 0 |
| 52 | 215 | 0 | 0 | Trace | Trace | 0 |
| 52 | 215 | 0 | 0 | Trace | Trace | 0 |
| 52 | 215 | 0 | 0 | Trace | Trace | 0 |
| 52 | 215 | 0 | 0 | Trace | Trace | 0 |

| | AVERAGE PORTION ml |
|---|---|
| **STOUT** | |
| Bottled | 250 |
| Extra | 287 |
| Guinness™ | 287 |
| Mackeson | 287 |
| | |
| **WINES** | |
| Champagne | 125 |
| Mulled wine | 125 |
| Red wine | 125 |
| Rosé, medium | 125 |
| White wine, dry | 125 |
| White wine, medium | 125 |
| White wine, sparkling | 125 |
| White wine, sweet | 125 |

| ENERGY kcal | ENERGY kJ | FAT g | SATURATED FAT g | PROTEIN g | CARBOHYDRATE g | FIBRE g |
|---|---|---|---|---|---|---|
| 93 | 390 | Trace | Trace | 1 | 10 | 0 |
| 112 | 468 | Trace | Trace | 1 | 6 | 0 |
| 86 | 362 | Trace | Trace | 1 | 4 | 0 |
| 103 | 439 | Trace | Trace | 1 | 13 | 0 |
| | | | | | | |
| 95 | 394 | 0 | 0 | 0 | 2 | 0 |
| 245 | 1028 | 0 | 0 | 0 | 32 | 0 |
| 85 | 354 | 0 | 0 | 0 | 0 | 0 |
| 89 | 368 | 0 | 0 | 0 | 3 | 0 |
| 83 | 344 | 0 | 0 | 0 | 1 | 0 |
| 93 | 385 | 0 | 0 | 0 | 4 | 0 |
| 93 | 384 | 0 | 0 | 0 | 6 | 0 |
| 118 | 493 | 0 | 0 | 0 | 7 | 0 |

© **Burger King** 66–67.
**Octopus Publishing Group Limited** 123 top right, /Jean Cazals 71 bottom right, 132 top left, /Stephen Conroy 101 top right, 127 bottom right, 130 bottom left, 131 top right, /Gus Filgate 52 bottom left, /Jeremy Hopley 8 top left, 59 bottom right, 132 bottom left, /David Jordan 8 bottom left, 16 top left, 58 bottom left, 76 bottom left, 77 top right, 87 top right, 102 bottom left, 131 bottom right, 133 bottom right, /Graham Kirk 126 bottom left, /Sandra Lane 86 bottom left, 114 bottom left, /William Lingwood 16 bottom left, 17 top right, 17 bottom right, 71 top right, 76 top left, 77 bottom right, 99 bottom right, 103 bottom right, 109 top right, /Neil Mersh 58 top left, 59 top left, /Peter Myers 52 top left, 130 top left, /Sean Myers 70 top left, 70 bottom left, /William Reavell 34 top left, 34 bottom left, 35 top right, 53 top right, 53 bottom right, 80 bottom left, 94 top left, 95 top right, 98 top left, 100 top left, 100 bottom left, 101 bottom right, 106 top left, 106 bottom left, 107 bottom right, 108 top left, 108 bottom left, 114 top left, 115 top right, 126 top left, 127 top right, 133 top right, /Simon Smith 80 top left, 81 top right, 81 bottom right, 95 bottom right, 102 top left, 103 top right, 107 top right, 122 top left, 122 bottom left, /Ian Wallace 9 top right, 9 bottom right, 86 top left, 87 bottom right, 94 bottom left, 99 top right, 109 bottom right, 115 bottom right, /Philip Webb 35 bottom right, 98 bottom left, 123 bottom right.
© **Kentucky Fried Chicken** 68–69.

**Commissioning Editor** Nicola Hill
**Editorial Director** Jane Birch
**Copy Editor** Cathy Lowne
**Executive Art Editor** Rozelle Bentheim
**Designer** Peter Gerrish
**Picture Researchers** Zoe Holtermann, Jennifer Veall
**Production Controller** Lucy Woodhead